BIRTHMARKS

A GUIDE TO
HEMANGIOMAS &
VASCULAR MALFORMATIONS

BIRTHMARKS

A GUIDE TO
HEMANGIOMAS &
VASCULAR MALFORMATIONS

BY

LINDA ROZELL SHANNON, M.S.

CONNIE MARSHALL, R.N., M.S.N.

WITH

MILTON WANER, M.D., MEDICAL EDITOR

WOMEN'S HEALTH PUBLISHING, INC.

Copyediting by Elizabeth Price Lindley
Cover design by Buster Hall
Printed in the United States of America

On the Cover: Christine Shannon at birth; at 11 months; and at $2\frac{1}{2}$ years of age, seven months after the removal of her hemangioma.

Women's Health Publishing, Inc.
1176 Angela Court, Ste. 103
Minden, NV 89423-8901

1-888-235-7947

ISBN # 0-9657056-0-9

Library of Congress Catalog Card Number # 97-60404

TABLE OF CONTENTS

PART II

VASCULAR MALFORMATIONS

PART III

PART IV

ACKNOWLEDGMENTS

Many wonderful people helped to make this book a reality. We would like to say a special thanks to :

The families of the children who shared their experiences and gave graciously of their time;

Our families for their patience, support, and understanding while we immersed ourselves in writing this book;

Joe Brogdon for the hours he spent interviewing families that provided invaluable insight into their personal experiences.

Diane Bussard, R.N., laser nurse at Arkansas Children's Hospital in Little Rock, for helping us coordinate the interview process with the families and for the TLC she gives to all who cross her path; and

Karla Hall who shared her expertise for the chapter on insurance and the appeals process.

Sherri Gunnell, R.N. and the Department of Otolaryngology at Arkansas Children's Hospital in Little Rock, for sharing their tracheostomy protocol;

Connie Marshall

My daughter, Christine Mary Shannon, the brave little soldier who endured her hemangioma and the surgery like a trooper; and to my mother, Theresa Rozell, who taught me to fight for my daughter's right to look normal;

Chuck Shannon, Christine's dad, and her grandmother, Charlotte Gallo, for their time and devotion to Christine enabling me to network with hundreds of "hemangioma" families; and

God for the gifts he has given me to help others.

James Y. Suen, M.D., chairman of the Department of Otolaryngology at the University of Arkansas for Medical Sciences, a friend and a brilliant surgeon who shaped my career and taught me so much. This book wouldn't have been possible without him.

PUBLISHER'S NOTE

The information, procedures, and suggestions included in this book are based on the experience, research, and practice of Milton Waner, M.D.

This book is not meant to supplant the advice or treatment of your physician. The treatment of hemangiomas and vascular malformations is in a state of change. The authors encourage you to share this information with your physician and discuss all options that are available regarding treatment of vascular lesions.

DEDICATION

This book is dedicated to all the children and families who endured, connected, nurtured, and supported each other through the trying times, and who rejoiced for each other during the process of treatment and healing. We hope this book provides a guiding light to the families who follow in your path.

INTRODUCTION

INTRODUCTION

Consider these statistics: Nearly 4 million children are born in the U.S. each year. Four hundred thousand children are born with a vascular birthmark. Ninety percent of these birthmarks disappear by 1 year of age. The remaining 10 percent will have a vascular birthmark that requires the opinion of a specialist.

If your child is one of the 40,000 babies born with a significant vascular birthmark, you already know the confusion and helplessness that comes with this problem as you look for information and help.

We have written this book for the parents and family of children with a vascular birthmark, whether it be a hemangioma ("strawberry"), or one of the vascular malformations such as a portwine stain, a venous malformation, or a lymphatic malformation. If you are an adult with a birthmark, you may also find this book valuable.

Much of the information in this book is new. Our hope is that it will contribute to changing the way vascular birthmarks are treated. We have drawn from many sources to produce this comprehensive book on hemangiomas and vascular malformations. We will give you accurate, up-to-date information, show you how to recognize the type of birthmark you or your child has, and provide suggestions on how to find the best treatment available.

The birth of a child with a vascular lesion can impose untold stress and pain on the whole family. You become forced to accept a challenge you didn't choose and to follow a path that is filled with fear and uncertainty. This period of time will test you in many ways. If you see this as a challenge and an opportunity to grow, the path will be less rocky.

Many children and their families have been down this road before you. We have drawn from their experiences as well as from many healthcare professionals. All have shared their expertise and experiences to make your journey less fearful and more hopeful. Throughout this book, we have made extensive use of illustrations and actual quotes from families that may mirror your feelings and experiences to show you that you're not alone.

We refer to children alternately as he and she, his and her. Since vascular hemangiomas affect three to five times as many girls as boys, references to the female gender are more heavily represented.

The information in this book will help you make educated decisions regarding the best treatment for your child. The color pictures on pages 81-88 are all patients of Milton Waner, M.D. and show some of the successful outcomes that are possible. This book is all about hope and healing and the fact that everyone has the right to look normal.

◆ ◆ ◆

BIRTHMARKS
PART I
HEMANGIOMAS

CHAPTER 1

CHAPTER 1

FACTS &

CLASSIFICATIONS

The diagnosis and treatment of vascular birthmarks continues to be a source of anxiety and confusion for both the families of the affected children and their healthcare providers.

Currently, there is no one single medical specialty dedicated to the diagnosis and treatment of vascular birthmarks. It makes the search for the "right" doctor extremely challenging. Commonly, the quest begins with the pediatrician and continues across the field of medical specialists from dermatologists to plastic surgeons and a multitude of sub-specialists. As you go from doctor to doctor, their diagnosis, philosophy of treatment, and the prognosis they offer often differs: One doctor might tell you your child's lesion is a hemangioma, while another says it's a vascular malformation. One doctor may say surgery might help but won't guarantee any results. Other doctors tell you it will go away in time; leave it alone. Their advice is meant to be reassuring, but your optimism may shrink as you watch the lesion grow.

"The first surgeon we saw turned down surgery on our daughter and said the risks were greater with surgery than with leaving it alone. The second surgeon said he would consider surgery, but could not promise a good outcome."

Your anxiety level increases as you discover your need to learn an entirely new language to try to understand what's happening to your child.

The language you hear is vaguely familiar but very confusing as you try to understand terms like lymphangioma, cystic hygroma and capillary-cavernous. No one seems to be even speaking the same language. Different doctors use different terms to describe the same lesion. The language problem is similar to the confusion it would cause if horticulturists referred to all flowers as roses. A rose is a flower, but not all flowers are roses. It's the same principle with vascular lesions.

It's common for *all* vascular lesions to be called hemangiomas. Hemangiomas are vascular lesions, but *all vascular lesions are not hemangiomas.* The terminology doctors previously used to define *vascular lesions* is in a state of much needed change. New, more precise methods of describing the different types of congenital lesions has replaced the old terminology that confused both the medical community and the lay public. The new terminology for hemangiomas and the old are listed below.

HEMANGIOMAS	
Old Term	**New Term**
Capillary strawberry	Superficial
Cavernous	Deep
Capillary-cavernous	Compound

What follows is the beginning of your education in the field of vascular lesions. Learn the language, learn the differences between the types of lesions and you're on your way to contributing to a correct diagnosis that will lead you to the correct treatment for your child's lesion.

THE BASICS

A hemangioma is *a benign,* blood-filled *tumor.* The word tumor is *not* to be confused with cancer. A hemangioma is not a cancer. Hemangiomas and vascular malformations are both vascular lesions. Many vascular malformations are mistakenly labeled as hemangiomas. We now know that not all vascular lesions are hemangiomas, and not all hemangiomas will go away.

> hemangioma-mass of blood vessels that increase in size and then shrink
>
> benign- non-cancerous
>
> tumor- a mass of tissue
>
> lesion-any abnormality in body tissue

"I have a granddaughter with two hemangiomas on her forehead, the size of golf balls...She has seen several specialists...her parents have been advised to wait until she is 5 years old and they will disappear. We believe that probably won't happen."

Hemangiomas and vascular malformations are vastly different from each other; they have different outcomes, and they are treated differently. To assure the best outcome in treating any congenital lesion (birthmark) the doctor has to first be sure what it is. The correct diagnosis leads to the correct treatment. The wrong diagnosis leads to treatment that is useless.

When working with your healthcare provider, remember that the field of congenital lesions is complicated and growing so rapidly that it's not always possible for each professional, not actively involved in the treatment of these lesions to be aware of all the most recent advances and treatments. Since you are seeking information and educating yourself to the available options, you may find yourself more knowledgeable in some respects than your primary healthcare provider regarding congenital lesions. If you find this to be true in your case, share your information and maintain a close working relationship with your primary physician who can help you find the resources and referrals you need.

> *"My son's physician was so grateful when I shared with him information I had received from one of the national support groups. He said that he had no idea there were so many new treatment options available."*

Education regarding the recent advances in the field of congenital lesions is important for both parents and the involved healthcare providers. With knowledge, the hope for the best outcome possible in each case can become a reality. Knowledge is the best way to replace helplessness and despair with hope and optimism.

THE FACTS

Hemangiomas are the most common benign tumor in infants. Fourteen in 100 children are born with a vascular birthmark, most are hemangiomas. Ten percent of these children require the opinion of a specialist while the others have insignificant hemangiomas or lesions which are small and located in an area covered by clothing.

Hemangiomas occur in up to 12 percent of all infants by one year of age. Twenty-three percent of those babies are very low birthweight (2.2 pounds or less). The reason for the high incidence of vascular lesions in low birthweight children is unknown.

Approximately 30 percent of hemangiomas are visible at birth. The majority of hemangiomas don't make their presence known until the first few weeks or even months after birth. The remaining 70 percent of lesions become visible between one and four weeks after birth. Rarely are hemangiomas fully grown at birth.

What actually causes hemangiomas is still a mystery. Some pieces of the puzzle are in place, but not all. The cause is *not* related to anything either you or your spouse did or didn't do during the pregnancy. No one is responsible for this condition. It's a birth defect. It just happened.

Hemangiomas are more common in whites. The darker the skin the less frequent the occurrence. The reason for this isn't known. One possible explanation is that there is an inherited cause for hemangiomas, but currently there is no evidence to support that theory.

"I have a hemangioma and I'm trying to get pregnant. I'm worried I could pass this along to my child."

Girls are three to five times more likely than boys to have a hemangioma. The hormone estrogen may play a significant role in the development of a hemangioma and its growth. Researchers recently discovered sites on the hemangioma cells that attract the hormone estrogen. As estrogen attaches to these receptor sites, it may stimulate the cells to increase in number. This finding may be an important clue as to how and why the tumor grows the way it does.

Hemangiomas may run in families, but a proven genetic or chromosomal link has yet to be found. Studies are under way to determine if there is a genetic link. The goal of research is to find a cause that can one day lead to prevention.

Many parents want to know if subsequent children are at risk for this type of birth defect. No one can say with great certainty that it won't happen, but it does appear that hemangiomas in subsequent births are rare.

7

Vascular lesions that appear in adults are often mistakenly called hemangiomas. Adults never develop hemangiomas; *only infants have true hemangiomas.* A vascular lesion appearing in adulthood is a vascular malformation or another type of internal or external vascular growth.

SIZE AND LOCATION

Hemangiomas are like people, they come in all shapes and sizes. Some are very small and hardly noticeable while others are large and very disfiguring. No one can predict how large any lesion will be, or why they all vary in size.

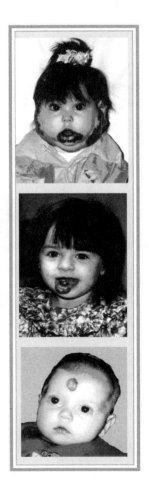

Eighty-three percent of hemangiomas occur on the head or neck, making these the most common sites. The remaining 17 percent occur on the trunk and limbs. Hemangiomas have favorite sites: between the eyes, the mouth area and the lower portion of the face. They may differ in size, but the lesions tend to occur in these same locations. Research is under way to determine why hemangiomas prefer certain sites over others.

In the early stage, a superficial hemangioma looks like a red spot while the deep hemangioma is more of a bluish spot.

8

The depth of the hemangioma determines which type of hemangioma it is. Collagen is the main protein component of our body's white fibrous tissues which includes skin, tendons, and connective tissue. If a lesion sits on top of the layer of collagen under the skin, it's called a superficial hemangioma. If the hemangioma lies under the collagen layer, it's considered a deep lesion.

SUPERFICIAL HEMANGIOMA

A superficial hemangioma is what used to be called a "strawberry" because some hemangiomas look like the skin of a strawberry. The appearance comes from millions of tiny dilated veins (telangiectasis) clumped and bunched together. The blood-filled veins give the hemangioma its red color.

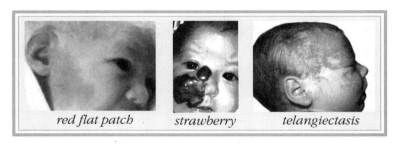

red flat patch   strawberry   telangiectasis

Most superficial hemangiomas will grow for 10 to 12 months and then begin the shrinking process called involution.

Hemangiomas can look like:

- a bright red, flat patch (macule) on the skin.
- a bright red, raised patch (papule) on the skin
- a cluster of tiny red veins (telangiectasis)

9

DEEP HEMANGIOMA

Due to the depth of the hemangioma, you may not notice it for many weeks or months after birth, but it's there and growing. By the time you can see the lesion, it's grown significantly. Unlike superficial hemangiomas, deep hemangiomas are bluish or flesh colored due to their depth. It feels firm and "rubbery" to the touch. When you press on the area, the color doesn't disappear.

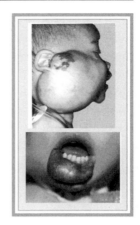

COMPOUND HEMANGIOMA

In some cases a child will have both a superficial and a deep hemangioma. While they are both hemangiomas, their location makes them different in the way they look. When both types of lesions appear together, it's called a compound hemangioma. With a lesion that has both a superficial and a deep component, the color may be a layered combination of red on top and blue below.

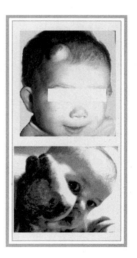

INTERNAL HEMANGIOMAS

Internal hemangiomas can form with no visible external signs, but the presence of multiple, *external* hemangiomas may indicate *internal* hemangioma(s). If there are six or more external hemangiomas, an ultrasound can verify if there are internal lesions. Hemangiomas can occur on organs such as the liver and cause yellow (jaundiced) skin with an enlarged abdomen, or even heart failure. On the intestines it may cause unexplained rectal bleeding, and in the respiratory system breathing problems can occur. If your child has external hemangiomas and develops any of these symptoms, ask your doctor to do an ultrasound, magnetic resonance imaging (MRI), or laryngoscopy to check for internal hemangiomas. Many children who have lesions affecting the lower face, called "beard" hemangiomas, develop breathing problems due to airway obstruction.

> Ultrasound- a visible moving image produced by the echo of sound waves.
>
> Magnetic Resonance Imaging- computer imaging of the body structures from magnetic field and radio frequency signals.
>
> laryngoscopy- procedure to visualize the larynx.

Internal hemangiomas can be very dangerous and should be treated promptly. Complications can be successfully overcome, if caught early or even prevented (see chapter 4).

◆ ◆ ◆

11

CHAPTER 1

CHAPTER 2
LIFE CYCLES & OUTCOMES

LIFE CYCLE OF A HEMANGIOMA

As your baby grows during the first year, so does the hemangioma. Somewhere between 10 and 14 months of age, the lesion begins to shrink and fade. The process can continue for 10 to 12 years. Some hemangiomas will completely disappear while others require corrective surgery. *Hemangiomas are the only vascular lesion to go through the process of growing and then shrinking.* All the other vascular lesions continue to enlarge all through life. *A lesion which is present at birth and continues to grow with the child beyond one year of age is most likely a vascular malformation, not a hemangioma.* Also, a lesion which is present at birth but does not actually appear or begin to grow for several years is undoubtedly a vascular malformation.

> proliferation-
> increase in cell
> division
>
> involution-
> process of
> shrinking in
> size

AGES AND STAGES

Hemangiomas *always* go through two stages: growth (proliferation) and shrinkage (involution). At different times during the first year of life, a hemangioma grows in size for a period of time and then lapses into a period of inactivity. During the first year many hemangiomas alternate between periods of growth and rest. Each hemangioma is unique with its own timetable for growing and resting.

During the growth period, most superficial hemangiomas become raised, shiny and bright red in color. The growth

13

results from cells multiplying and forming the dense network of tiny new blood vessels. During the growth process, the cells are plump. The hemangioma feels warm to the touch and can swell when the baby is upset or sick. Un-

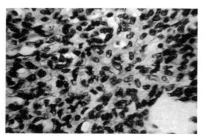

Process of Cell Growth

doubtedly, there is some discomfort to the child as the cells within the lesion multiply. As they expand in size, the skin stretches making it tender and tight. Luckily, the skin usually stretches enough to accommodate the increased growth of the lesion. Occasionally, where the growth is particularly rapid, the skin may tear from the tension leaving an open sore called an *ulcer* (see page 37). During its rest period, the superficial hemangioma fades to a more dusky rose color.

For most hemangiomas, there are two growth cycles: the Primary Growth Cycle lasting from birth to two months of age, and the Secondary Growth Cycle starting around the fourth month and lasting for six-to-eight additional months. Remember, each hemangioma has its own timetable. Some follow the two cycles of growth while others continue to grow steadily throughout the first year of life.

Between the tenth and twelfth month, most hemangiomas stop growing. It's important to understand these growth cycles because you can get a false sense of security when it appears that the hemangioma has stopped growing at the end of the Primary Growth Cycle. This rest period can last for months and give the false impression that treatment isn't needed.

Some hemangiomas are late bloomers and skip the first cycle of growth in the early weeks of life. They don't begin their growth phase until the four-to-six month period. Within this one year time frame, each hemangioma seems to have a timetable of

14

its own. No one knows what signals the lesion to wind down this phase of its life cycle and begin its next phase. It's important to follow the growth and rest cycle of each particular lesion to help determine the most effective treatment.

INVOLUTION

By the end of the first year, the hemangioma completes its growth phase and begins a longer cycle of shrinking. The cells within the hemangioma, the culprits in the growth process, reach the end of this phase of their life cycle, lose their plumpness and deflate like an airless inner tube. As the lesion shrinks, the blood vessels become more prominent.

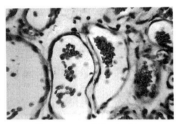

Process of Shrinking

It's possible that there are two types of regression cycles to hemangiomas: a Rapid Regression Cycle and a Slow Regression Cycle. With the rapid regressors, 60 percent completely shrink by age six, but 40 percent of these lesions still require some form of corrective surgery. The rapid regressor hemangiomas usually make a noticeable change by the time the child is two to four years old. The lesion will be smaller, noticeably lighter in color, and softer in texture. By this stage, it should be possible to tell in which group your child's lesion belongs.

Half of hemangiomas are slow regressors. These lesions persist for up to 10 or 12 years, but only 20 percent completely shrink. The remaining 80 percent need corrective surgery.

A word of advice: when you see the lesion every day, it's difficult to notice change until it's significant. Get to know the lesion as well as you know your baby. Keep a monthly log and record the growth pattern of the lesion with a photo and measurements. Don't be afraid to measure it with a tape measure. This information will be very helpful to the physician planning treatment.

Slow or Rapid Regressors

By age two to four, the slow regressor lesion will have little or no change in size. It may be lighter in color, but the size is usually unchanged. Usually, if no change in size is seen by age two to four, you can consider it a slow regressor. This information is important because it may determine which hemangiomas require active intervention. Remember, 60 percent of all hemangiomas require some form of corrective surgery. Eighty percent of the slow regressors and 40 percent of the rapid regressors need corrective surgery.

The lower lip is a common area for slow regression. A large lesion in this area is disfiguring. The lesion stretches and elongates the lip creating problems with eating and talking. Active intervention is usually necessary.

Knowing whether the type of regression is slow or rapid is significant to the treatment of the remaining lesion. With a rapid regressor, you may be able to postpone corrective surgery to make sure it's necessary. If the lesion is a slow regressor, showing no signs of change by age two to four, early corrective surgery should begin early to prevent further psychosocial trauma.

All hemangiomas, if they are truly hemangiomas, shrink. The big question is: how much? The term involution means different things to different people. Ideally, at the completion of the involution stage, the hemangioma *completely* disappears. Unfortunately, that's not true for all hemangiomas.

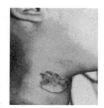

Involuted Hemangioma

16

While most hemangiomas will be gone by the time the child is 10 years old, the result will not be perfect. The hemangioma may be gone, but the lesion may still require some form of corrective surgery. In reality, for those hemangiomas that complete involution by age six, 40 percent of the cases still have very visible scarring and telangiectasis. When a hemangioma doesn't complete its involution phase by age six, 80 percent of cases are left with a significant deformity.

The involution phase of the hemangioma takes from two to twelve years. It's difficult to predict precisely how long the involution process will last for each lesion. Here are some average spans of involution:

- By five years of age, 50 percent of hemangiomas complete their involution phase.

- By seven years of age, 70 percent resolve.

- The remaining cases take three to five years *longer* to complete their involution process.

How Do You Know It's Shrinking?

There are some tangible signs the lesion is in the involution phase. You know it's shrinking:

- when it's less tender (painful) and softer to the touch.

- when the hemangioma doesn't get bigger when your child cries.

- when a superficial hemangioma turns from a bright red to a dark, deep maroonish hue, or to a grayish hue.

17

OUTCOMES

Once the involution (shrinking) phase begins, a superficial hemangioma fades to a dull maroon hue and becomes much softer to the touch. Later, it becomes gray and mottled from the center of the lesion outward. Over a period of years, the gray gradually turns to a very light flesh color. A deep hemangioma, on the other hand, doesn't have a color change, but becomes softer as the involution process proceeds..

A large superficial hemangioma upon complete regression, may have a wrinkled crepe-paper-like appearance (epidermal atrophy) not unlike someone who lost a lot of weight quickly and has stretch marks. The problem comes from the loss of collagen and elastin. Collagen is the substance that gives skin both its thickness and smooth appearance and elastin its elasticity. The growth of the hemangioma also results in the destruction of elastin. During the active growth stage, the hemangioma displaces collagen. When the lesion shrinks, there is no collagen to support the skin and fill in the gap; the skin is loose and wrinkled. The color of the affected skin may be slightly lighter than the child's skin tone. Superficial hemangiomas also leave red veins. The excess skin can be removed surgically, resurfaced with a CO_2, and the veins removed with laser therapy.

If the hemangioma ulcerated or bled excessively, there will always be a white scar where the ulceration or bleeding occurred. There is no way to prevent this scarring, but it can be treated with corrective surgery or skin resurfacing.

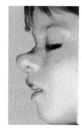

Hemangiomas at the tip of the nose tend to be disfiguring and slow regressors. The lesion pushes the nasal tip cartilages apart. This splaying effect remains even after involution is completed. Corrective surgery works well to repair the problem.

Deep hemangiomas may leave a contour type deformity, a lumpy area under the skin made up of deposits of fibro-fatty tissue. Surgical removal eliminates this problem.

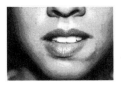

Compound hemangiomas leave varying degrees of both the superficial and deep lesions: crepe-like excess skin, red veins, and fibro-fatty tissue. All these problems can be treated.

> **Untreated Hemangioma Outcomes**
>
> *Superficial:* wrinkled crepe-like appearance, red veins
> *Deep:* contour deformity, fibro fatty tissue
> *Compound:* a combination of all of the above

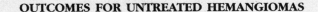

OUTCOMES FOR UNTREATED HEMANGIOMAS

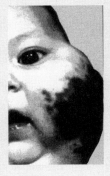
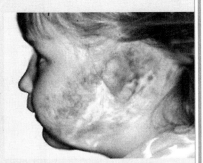

Giant parotid hemangioma involuted at age six years with scarring and destruction of the ear cartilage.

OUTCOMES FOR UNTREATED HEMANGIOMAS

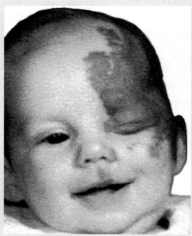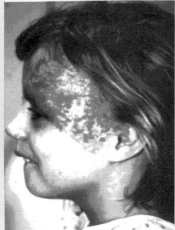

Extensive, hemangioma from proliferation to involution at five years of age with residual blood vessels (telangiectasis).

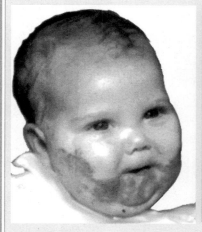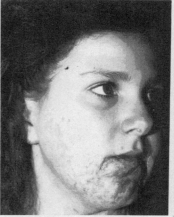

Extensive, hemangioma from proliferation to involution. Outcome at age 16 years with scarring and crepe-like skin.

OUTCOMES OF TREATED HEMANGIOMAS

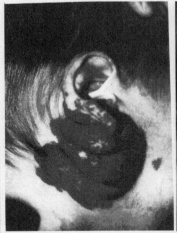 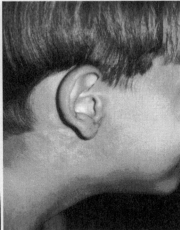

Three year old with extensive parotid hemangioma before and after laser treatment.

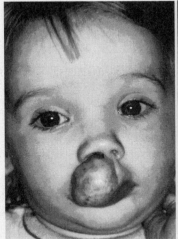 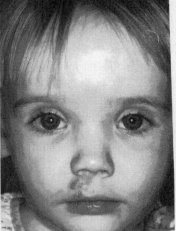

Eighteen month old with lip hemangioma before and after excision.

OUTCOMES OF TREATED HEMANGIOMAS

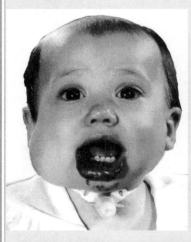 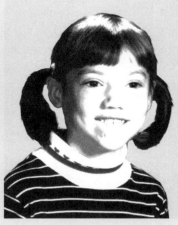

Six month old with extensive hemangioma of the lower lip and airway that required a tracheostomy. At five years of age after multiple laser treatments and two surgeries.

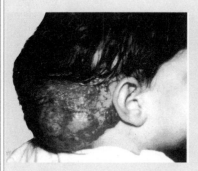 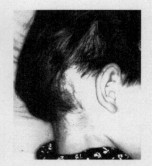

Eighteen month old with extensive hemangioma resulting in heart failure requiring treatment and surgical excision of the lesion.

CHAPTER 3

ADVANCES IN
TREATMENT

TO TREAT OR NOT TO TREAT

When you go looking for help with your child's hemangioma, the process is often as confusing as the condition itself. Not everyone agrees on the best approach.

> *"Our daughter has many large hemangiomas on her face and lips. The first doctor we took her to did laser surgery on the outside of her lip. The second doctor we took her to said that she was not concerned about the hemangiomas on my daughter's lip but rather the ones in her mouth. She said they could affect her teeth as well as cause other problems. I was told that we should "wait and see."*

Many physicians still advise parents to let the hemangioma resolve on its own and forego treatment. This policy, known as "benign neglect," began over 50 years ago when a physician discovered that the lesions would shrink over time and determined they were best left alone. This "wait and see" or "benign neglect" approach is still being taught in medical schools and reinforced in medical textbooks. *It's time for a change.* Fortunately, a growing number of prominent physicians across the country, who are actively involved in treating hemangiomas, have recognized the positive results, both physically and psychologically, of early intervention.

Here are some issues to consider when making the decision to treat or not to treat:

EMOTIONAL EFFECTS

The psychosocial trauma suffered by a child with a disfiguring hemangioma is immense and cannot be overlooked. The pain and stress of the family having to deal with this problem is equally damaging.

> *"My son has a hemangioma that is being treated....It's very painful to go shopping with him and watch everyone stare. I really want my beautiful baby boy to have this all taken care of before school."*

A child develops self-awareness at eighteen to twenty-four months of age. Give careful thought to the emotional and psychological impact to your child who has to live with a cosmetic deformity that may be present for as long as 12 years. At the end of those years, it's possible the cosmetic results would be both disappointing and unacceptable(see outcomes section). Remember, 80 percent of lesions not healed by age six leave a significant deformity. Even 40 percent of those lesions that heal by age six still have unacceptable cosmetic results. The goal is to help your child look normal before starting school. Even a small physical scar is preferable to a deep emotional one.

> *"I am convinced that if he could speak, he would ask to have it taken care of. When I see interviews of older children who are slightly or greatly disfigured, I hear only how happy they are to look "more normal."*

RECENT ADVANCES AND TREATMENTS

In the last 10 years, the advances in treating vascular lesions have been enormous. Lasers can selectively destroy the abnormal blood vessels of a hemangioma. Drugs can inhibit the growth of the cells while the thermoscalpels and special lasers offers almost bloodless surgery.

24

Not all hemangiomas require treatment, but more than half will require some form of corrective surgery. There is a strong case for doing the necessary corrective work as soon as possible, especially before the child starts school.

Types of Treatment Available

Since each stage in the life cycle of the hemangioma is unique, there are different types of treatment available that can be used in more than one stage. It's really best to plan treatment according to the *stage* of the lesion.

- During the early growth phase of the lesion, aggressive intervention aims at complete elimination of the lesion or significant slowing of the growth.

- During the intermediate period of 12 months to $3\frac{1}{2}$ years of age, it's a "wait and see" period. If the lesion begins to shrink rapidly, a favorable outcome is likely, and treatment may not be needed. If the lesion is shrinking slowly, treatment should be started since 80 percent of these lesions need corrective surgery. The benefits of correcting the lesions before the child starts school outweigh any benefits from a period of benign neglect.

- The late phase of involution calls for aggressive intervention starting from the age of three and a half onward to complete correction before school age.

Choosing the best treatment is a complex process needing careful consideration with a plan to individualize treatment according to your child's needs. An accurate diagnosis and a physician actively involved in the field of vascular lesions is the critical first step to an effective treatment plan.

> *"We found a doctor who had experience in operating on children with hemangiomas. Today our daughter is doing very well."*

As a parent, you can play an important role in assuring a correct diagnosis that will lead to the best treatment outcome. Ask yourself these questions:

- When did you first notice the lesion?
- Has it grown?
- Is it shrinking?

If the lesion was not visible at birth but appeared during the first few weeks after birth, it's probably a hemangioma. If it grows during the first year of life and begins shrinking after the first year, it's definitely a hemangioma.

The three types of treatment options for a hemangioma are:

- Drug Therapy
   steroids-oral or injections directly into the lesion
   (intralesional)
   alpha-interferon (daily injections)
- Laser Surgery
- Surgical Removal

Effective treatment for a hemangioma depends upon several factors such as the child's age, the stage of growth, and the phase of involution of the lesion. Some types of treatment work best in the early stage of growth and others during late growth.

TREATMENT DURING EARLY GROWTH STAGE

During the early growth stage, the lesion is active and aggressive. If the cells are closer to the surface, they're more accessible to treatment with a laser.

Laser surgery is one of the most exciting and effective treatments now available. With hemangiomas, the laser's intense beam of light penetrates the skin without affecting it. The light is selectively attracted to and absorbed by the red blood cells. No other structures are affected. The energy is converted to heat which destroys the blood vessels from within. Unfortunately, the depth of penetration of the laser is very superficial, partly because of the high ability of the red blood cells to absorb the light. Treating a hemangioma with a laser is a little like peeling an onion: It's done one layer at a time. It's common to have multiple laser treatments to totally remove the lesion. Laser surgery is not painless. Anesthesia, either general or intravenous sedation, should be considered as part of the treatment plan. If your child's hemangioma is large, discuss the options with your doctor.

There are several types of lasers that can be used to treat hemangiomas. The lasers that generate too much heat and destroy much more than the targeted blood vessels are not the lasers of choice. The laser that can safely do the job is the flashlamp pumped dye laser (see chapter 8).

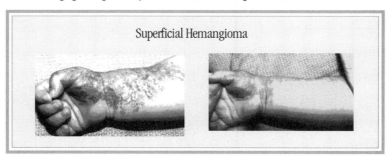
Superficial Hemangioma

Flashlamp pumped dye lasers work effectively on a flat, superficial lesion still in the early growing stage. Treatment begins at the earliest sign of the lesion and is repeated at four-to-six week intervals until the lesion disappears. A child with this type of lesion may need as many as six treatments to complete the healing process. The laser can completely re-move a superficial hemangioma in the early growth stage. In some cases, removing the superficial lesion uncovers a previ-ously undetected deep hemangioma. With a deep lesion, the laser can't penetrate deeply enough to have any effect. A disfiguring deep hemangioma should be treated with a course of oral steroids if the child is under 1 year of age. If the lesion is well localized and not too large, an intralesional injection may be beneficial (see next section).

TREATMENT DURING LATE GROWTH STAGE

In this late stage of growth, the lesion is often too deep and thick for the type of laser therapy that works well with superficial lesions in the early growth stage.

STEROIDS

Steroid drugs such as cortisone reduce inflammation. For reasons unknown, they also shrink growing hemangiomas. Dur-ing your child's first year of life when the hemangioma is still growing, an oral steroid (Prednisone) may help shrink the lesion. *Steroids will have no effect if the lesion is no longer in the growth phase. For this reason, they are rarely given after 1 year of age.*

Prednisone treatment continues over the course of four weeks, and the dose is then slowly decreased over the follow-ing two months. The critical factor with steroids is giving a dose that will work most effectively. Recent studies advise giving the child 3-5 milligrams (mg) per kilogram (kg) of body weight with the drugs Zantac and Propulsid (or their equivalent) to prevent stomach irritation and acid reflux.

The key to steroid therapy: Give the appropriate dose to achieve the desired effect, and continue the steroid during the growth phase of the hemangioma, or until about the seventh month when the growth slows. Within seven to ten days, it should be apparent if the drug is having the desired effect. If the lesion isn't shrinking within a week, the dose should be tapered over a week and discontinued (see appendix 2).

If the lesions responds to the steroid by shrinking, we recommend continuing the full dose for at least 3-4 weeks and then decrease it gradually over an 8-10 week period. *The goal is to slow the growth and shrink the lesion as much as possible until the growth phase is over.* A smaller lesion is obviously easier to treat.

Unfortunately, not all hemangiomas respond to steroids in the same way. Some lesions will begin to grow again when the steroid is decreased. If that happens, the full dose can be given again for 2 weeks and then start decreasing the dosage. If the lesion grows again, the process is repeated until it no longer resumes the growth process when the drug is decreased.

If your child receives steroids, you must be prepared to:

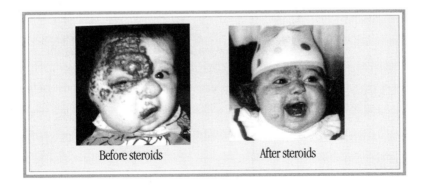

Before steroids   After steroids

- have her on steriods for months if necessary.
- have her monitored weekly by her primary care physician.
- delay immunizations until steroid treatment is discontinued, especially live vaccines such as polio.
- *give her an acid inhibiting drug such as Zantac to counter the gastric irritation.*

The potential side effects from oral steroids are :

- temporary slowing in physical growth
- swelling of face (moon face)
- behavioral changes such as irritability and crying
- peptic ulcer
- loss of appetite
- increased risk of certain infections

Fortunately, few of these problems occur. The most common side effect is gastric irritation, irritability and the moon face (see appendix 2). *The side effects listed above disappear when the drug is stopped.*

Helpful Hint:

Some children don't like the taste of the syrup. You put it in and it comes right out. If your child spits out or doesn't tolerate the syrup form of steroid treatment, talk to your doctor about switching to the tablet form. Crush the tablet and mix it in cereal, ice cream, yogurt or pudding. It's critical she gets her daily dosage.

Some physicians prefer injecting the lesion with steroids to shrink the hemangioma. This technique works when the lesion is small and well localized. The lesion may need two treatments spaced six-to-eight weeks apart.

Some people feel there are no real advantages to injection over the oral method of treatment. The injection technique is painful. Sedation or general anesthesia should be considered.

Once you inject the steroid, you can't take it back. With the oral route, you can discontinue the drug or reduce the dosage, so there's more finite control. Injecting the steroid doesn't avoid the systemic side effects of the drug. Injecting an upper eyelid lesion carries some risks that can result in blindness. Discuss these potential problems with your doctor before proceeding with steroid injections.

If the lesion fails to respond to steroids, either surgery for the deep hemangioma and laser therapy for the superficial hemangioma is a good approach when the lesion is particularly large, growing rapidly, or disfiguring. Magnetic Resonance Imaging (MRI), another new, immensely valuable tool, visualizes the exact extent of the lesion before surgery so the surgeon can plan the best approach to treatment. If surgery seems the best approach, choose a skilled surgeon to do this delicate task (see chapter 7). This is not an operation for the faint-hearted or unskilled. The possibilities for excessive bleeding are obvious. Even with the newer technologies such as the thermal scalpel and certain types of lasers to minimize blood loss during surgery, only a very skilled, surgeon with experience in this type of surgery should do it.

Interferon

Interferon is an anti-viral drug that was accidently found to shrink vascular tumors. The drug is given just under the skin (subcutaneously) by injection. It shrinks the tumor as

31

Prednisone does. The usual dose is 3 million units per meter squared of body surface area, given daily for several months.

High doses of steroids should be given before using interferon. *If the lesion responds (shrinks, lightens or softens) to steroid treatment, it may not be necessary to give interferon.*

A small number of patients develop a permanent spasticity from interferon. It should only be given if:

- steroid treatment fails.
- there are no other options.
- the condition is life or sight-threatening such as Kassabach-Merritt syndrome, cardiac failure, airway obstruction, and visual obstruction.

> Interferon dosage
> Calculating Example:
> height = 27 inches
> weight = 11 pounds
>
> Convert inches to cms and pounds to kgs.
> 27 x 2.54 = 68.5 cms
> 11 lbs divided by 2.2=5kg
>
> Formula for dosage:
> $$^{m2}\frac{[ht(cm) \times wt(kg)}{3600}$$
>
> 68.5 X 5 kg = 342.5
> 342.5 divided by 3600=
> .095
> 3 million units X .095=
> 285,000 units/day

TREATMENT DURING EARLY INVOLUTION

Between eight and fourteen months of age, the lesion completes its stage of growth and begins involuting (shrinking). By age $3\frac{1}{2}$ it becomes obvious if the lesion is shrinking slowly or rapidly.

A lesion that is rapidly shrinking has a 60 percent chance of not causing disfigurement. In this case, it's preferable to adopt the "wait and see" approach. If the defect is large and has a superficial component, laser therapy can remove it. Forty percent of rapid regressors may still require minor corrective surgery to remove

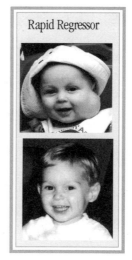
Rapid Regressor

residual skin or to correct a deformity which may have resulted from the hemangioma.

If you make the decision to treat the hemangioma, we suggest that superficial lesions should be treated with a laser, deep lesions should be excised, and compound lesions treated with both excision and laser.

Timing of Treatment

By age three, it's apparent if the lesion is regressing slowly and treatment will need to be done at some point. Why wait until the child is six years old and already in school? If you know you're going to need to do some type of corrective surgery, why wait? If you start by age three, the treatments can be completed before your child starts school.

TREATMENT DURING LATE INVOLUTION

Frequently, in the late stages of shrinking, the lesion will leave a web of spider veins, excess skin, thin, tissue paper-like skin and fibro-fatty tissue. All of these can be treated and removed. The flashlamp pumped dye laser removes the spider veins. Skin resurfacing with a carbon dioxide (CO_2) laser removes the excess skin on the face and neck, and tightens collagen to smooth the skin. Any fibro-fatty tissue can be removed surgically.

The most effective treatment to correct a hemangioma and its disfiguring effects requires the teamwork of parents and experienced healthcare professionals. The most appropriate treatment depends upon the type, age and stage of the lesion. New modalities of treatment and a keener knowledge of the life cycles of hemangiomas give great hope for great outcomes. *Everyone deserves to look normal.*

◆ ◆ ◆

LIFE CYCLE OF A TYPICAL HEMANGIOMA

LESION PRESENTS AT BIRTH OR IN EARLY INFANCY

↓

GROWS DURING FIRST YEAR OF LIFE

red in color   *blue in color*

↓   ↓

raised or flat   *firm and rubbery*

↓   ↓

SUPERFICIAL   DEEP

HEMANGIOMA   HEMANGIOMA

↓

SHRINKS

CHAPTER 4

POSSIBLE COMPLICATIONS

There are some important possible complications involving hemangiomas. Read the following and become familiar with the important symptoms that will help avoid emergencies.

ULCERATION

The most common complication of a superficial hemangioma is ulceration. As it grows, the hemangioma challenges the ability of the skin to stretch; if the skin can't accommodate the growth of the hemangioma, it splits open and creates an ulcer. It's not unusual for the hemangioma to split and begin bleeding spontaneously from even the slightest bump. The split skin races to close and repair the tear. At the same time, the lesion is growing faster than the skin can repair the damage. As a result, the ulcer may not heal for months.

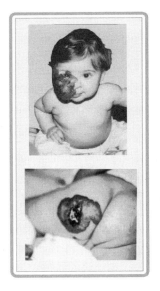

Infection is common with an ulcer, particularly on the lip, the perianal, and genital areas. When the ulcer comes in contact with urine and feces, it's painful. It's especially important to treat any diaper area hemangiomas as soon as they are diagnosed to prevent pain, further ulceration and tissue destruction. Ulcerated hemangiomas are often treated with a flashlamp pumped dye laser.

A topical antibiotic may be applied to the ulcer. Long-term use of topical antibiotics always poses a risk of the skin becoming hypersensitive. Bacitracin and Polysporin have less risk of hypersensitivity with long-term use.

AIRWAY OBSTRUCTION

A baby's airway extends from the tip through the back of the nose (nasopharynx), the back of the throat (oropharynx), through to the voice box (larynx) to the windpipe (trachea). In the chest, the windpipe splits with a tube going to each lung. A hemangioma can obstruct the airway *anywhere* in this route. Babies naturally breathe through their noses during the first few weeks of life. If a lesion obstructs both nasal airways during this time, it's a life-threatening situation. It's possible but unlikely for a hemangioma to obstruct both nasal passages. The goal of treatment is to shrink the cause of obstruction and relieve the breathing difficulty. Aggressive intervention with steroids, and, in some cases, laser surgery can often prevent a rapidly growing hemangioma from obstructing the airway.

Two of the most serious problems associated with nasal hemangiomas are destruction of cartilage, either the nostril or the nasal septum, and displacement of the cartilage that forms the nasal tip. As the hemangioma grows in this area, it pushes the cartilages that form the nasal tip apart. When the hemangioma finally shrinks, the nose is disfigured. It seems best to excise the nasal tip hemangioma as soon as possible.

PHARYNGEAL HEMANGIOMAS

Pharyngeal hemangiomas are usually associated with a particular pattern involving the lower third of the face that stretches from in front of one ear to the chin and then to the other side of the face. This type of hemangioma obstructs the airway sometime during the first six months of life. A child with a pharyngeal hemangioma that is obstructing will have symptoms of noisy breathing during inhalation. Aggressive intervention with steroids to shrink the lesion is the first line of treatment. If the obstruction isn't relieved, a tracheostomy would have to be done. See chapter 8.

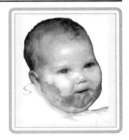

SUB-GLOTTIC HEMANGIOMAS

A hemangioma affecting the larynx may be above or below the vocal cords, or involve the vocal cords themselves. This type of hemangioma can appear within the first eight weeks after birth and will obstruct the airway far quicker than a pharyngeal hemangioma will. The hemangioma actually begins to grow inside the airway and obstructs breathing. The child develops a croupy, barking cough with noisy breathing on both inhalation and exhalation. Most laryngeal hemangiomas, that don't respond to aggressive steroid treatment, require a tracheostomy so the child can breathe until the hemangioma involutes to the point it no longer obstructs the airway (see chapter 8). If the hemangioma is diagnosed early enough, aggressive steroid or interferon treatment may prevent the need for tracheostomy.

VISUAL

The retina doesn't complete its development until some time after birth. If you block one eye for a period of even five days during this time, the child will stop using that eye and the nerve fibers don't develop. The condition is called "deprivation amblyopia" which will lead to blindless in the affected eye. Any hemangioma that obstructs the visual field during this period of development, and persists for longer than one week, will result in deprivation amblyopia. It's the commonest cause of blindness in the developed world.

If the hemangioma doesn't obstruct the visual field, but rests within the eyelid, the anatomy of the cornea of the eye is altered and this results in astigmatism. If the astigmatism is severe, the child will favor the other eye and is at risk for developing amblyopia. Hemangiomas on the eyelid that result in astigmatism can be 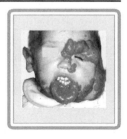 treated. Surgical removal or reduction in size with steroids will result in correction of astigamtism if it's done early enough. Many ophthamologists use intralesional injections of a steroid for treatment. The injections may need to be repeated to obtain a lasting effect.

If the hemangioma is growing and looks as if it will obstruct the visual axis, this is an emergency. The hemangioma can be treated with a course of steroids to reduce the size and relieve the obstruction to the child's vision. If the steroid treatment fails, interferon may be used and surgical removal may need to be considered.

RARE BLEEDING DISORDERS

KASSABACH-MERRITT SYNDROME

Platelets are one of the components in the blood that helps clotting. With Kassabach-Merritt syndrome, the hemangioma traps and destroys platelets so the blood's ability to clot is compromised. As the hemangioma grows, it traps more and more platelets. The body's ability to clot decreases. Spontaneous hemorrhage becomes likely. This is a very serious complication and fatal in 30 to 40 percent of cases.

The type of hemangioma that causes Kassabach-Merritt syndrome appears in the first few weeks after birth. The most common sites are the face and neck (parotid) areas. This hemangioma seems to be very different from the start. Here are some important early signs:

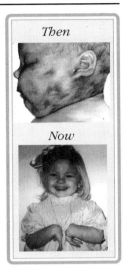

Then

Now

- swelling of skin overlying the hemangioma.
- reddish and purple bruises within the skin.

Any very large hemangioma should be suspect for Kassabach-Merritt syndrome. Blood levels should be checked if a child has an aggressive, large hemangioma prior to six months of age. The treatment of the syndrome should be managed by a hematologist or a physician experienced in treating these lesions. The child needs hospitalization and careful monitoring until they are stable. Steroids are usually started with the maximum dose given for up to four weeks and then tapered very slowly over 2-to-3 months. Interferon may also be used. If the lesion responds to interferon, the physician may want to try and discontinue the steroids and just use the interferon. Since interferon has the potential to cause permanent spasticity, it should be used with caution. If the situation is life-threatening, the benefits of interferon treatment outweigh the risks.

DISSEMINATED INTRAVASCULAR COAGULATION (DIC)

With this extremely rare bleeding disorder, the blood platelets and other clotting factors are depleted by a large blood clot in the growing hemangioma. This blood clot grows until, eventually, all the platelets and other clotting factors are depleted. Heparin is given to try and stop the clot from growing, but it doesn't always work. Because DIC is such a catastrophic condition, death often results.

HIGH OUPUT CARDIC FAILURE

Heart failure of this type is usually caused by a very large, solitary hemangioma on the head and neck area, or multiple systemic hemangiomas on the liver and intestines. This problem can occur anytime during proliferation or early involution. The early symptom of this problem can appear as an infant that fails to eat well and does not gain weight (failure to thrive).

The hemangioma shunts blood from the arterial to the venous side, putting a strain on the heart which has to work harder and harder to pump the blood. Over time, the heart enlarges so it can pump more efficiently. The heart is a muscle, and it can only enlarge to a certain point. When that point is reached, it can't compensate or continue to function. If the heart doesn't pump the blood out fast enough, it starts backing up in lungs. The child becomes short of breath, fluids stay in the tissues appearing as a pot belly with swelling (edema). Fluid also collects in the lungs so these children are especially susceptible to chest infections. Without treatment, 40 to 50 percent of these children die.

Treatment entails eliminating the cardiac failure with drugs or surgically removing the hemangioma. Before any surgical excision is tried, aggressive steroid treatment should be used first, and then interferon if steroids fail. Only a surgeon skilled in removing lesions around the facial nerves should perform this type of surgery.

♦ ♦ ♦

HEMANGIOMAS:

- always grow during the first year of life.
- are bright red during growth phase.
- turn dusky rose color during rest phase.
- have Primary Growth Phase from birth to 2-to-3 months of age.
- have Secondary Growth Phase from either 4-to-6 months of age.
- may have their own growth and rest cycle time tables.
- always shrink after the first year.
- take two to twelve years to completely involute.
- have two types of involution cycles: rapid and slow. Sixty percent of Rapid Regressors involute by age 6. *Forty percent of these need corrective surgery.*
- that regress slowly, need *early corrective surgery.*

TREATMENT RECOMMENDATIONS

Early Growth Phase:

If superficial, use laser to eliminate the lesion completely.

If deep, use steroids to eliminate completely or stunt growth. Surgery is sometimes considered for complicated or severely disfiguring lesions.

Intermediate Period

At 12 months to $3\frac{1}{2}$ years of age, if lesion is shrinking slowly, start corrective surgery which may entail a combination of laser and surgical correction.

Late Phase Involution

Start aggressive intervention at $3\frac{1}{2}$ years of age to complete correction before school age.

BIRTHMARKS

PART II

VASCULAR
MALFORMATIONS

CHAPTER 5

CHAPTER 5

CLASSIFICATIONS

VASCULAR MALFORMATION

THE BASICS

Vascular malformations are an abnormal cluster of blood vessels that occur during fetal development. Since vascular malformations are a developmental abnormality, they're always present at birth, but may not be visible until days, weeks or years after birth. The abnormality occurs as commonly in males as females, as opposed to hemangiomas which are much more common in females. Vascular malformations are very different from hemangiomas. How they differ is very important:

Unlike hemangiomas, vascular malformations do not proliferate. The cells within the vascular malformation do not increase in number as they do in a hemangioma. Instead, the size of the existing cells and blood vessels in the vascular malformation expand, a condition called hypertrophy. Unlike a hemangioma, the vascular malformation doesn't usually grow rapidly during the first year of life. The growth is normally slow and steady, although some vascular malformations grow much more rapidly than others.

> Vascular- refers to blood vessels.
>
> Vein- blood vessel that carries blood back to the heart.
>
> Venous- refers to veins
>
> Venular- small vein
>
> Arteriovenous- refers to abnormal movement of blood directly from an artery to a vein, bypassing the normal route.
>
> Capillary- smallest blood vessels.
>
> Lymphatic- thin-walled vessel that collects excess tissue fluid.

The lesions that grow more rapidly than normal are called "high-grade" malformations. Those lesions that expand more slowly are called "low-grade" malformations.

A vascular malformation, in contrast to a hemangioma, does not shrink over time. This is an important point, especially when you're trying to decide whether a lesion is a hemangioma or a vascular malformation. Initially, it can be confusing since both lesions can be seen at birth, and some vascular malformations can look like a deep hemangioma. A correct diagnosis is important because the treatment of vascular malformations is different from that of hemangiomas.

> *"We saw a series of doctors...They did a number of very painful steroid injections in our daughter's lip. Not only was the diagnosis incorrect, but what he was doing was fruitless!"*

TYPES OF VASCULAR MALFORMATIONS

Midline Venular Malformations

Midline venular malformations were previously known as capillary malformations. They are what grandma used to call "stork bites" and "angel kisses." The names are very benign and so are the malformations. They're flat lesions with a light pink color that usually fades during the first year of life.

Angel kisses are always in the midline area such as the upper eyelids, forehead, the brow area between the eyes (glabella), and the upper lip.

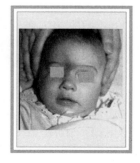

Stork bites occur on the nape of the neck and the middle of the lower (sacral) region of the back. Occasionally, a lesion in the sacral area may indicate there's an underlying defect in the spinal column. Stork bites and angel kisses, by themselves, are not associated with spinal defects; but a lesion on the midline, or in the lower back area, should be examined by a doctor. Sometimes, midline venular malformations are mistaken for portwine stains. Unlike portwine stains, these lesions are always midline, and very rarely do they thicken and darken like a portwine stain.

Venular Malformation (Portwine Stain)

A portwine stain (PWS) is another name for a venular malformation. Portwine stains are always present at birth, but may not be noticed for the first few days. In the past, these lesions were erroneously referred to as capillary hemangiomas, but that term is confusing and shouldn't be used. A portwine stain will occur in .3% of births, and the lesion occurs equally among males and females, unlike hemangiomas.

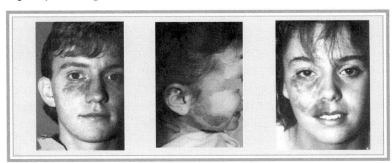

The cause of a portwine stain is most likely a deficiency or absence in the nerve supply to the blood vessels of the affected area. These nerves control the diameter of the blood vessels. If the nerves are absent, the vessels continue to dilate and enlarge. The location of the birthmark seems to follow the distribution of certain cutaneous (skin) nerves. For example, the trigeminal nerve is the main sensory nerve for the skin of the face, which is a common site for portwine stains. Some portwine stains cover a large surface area; others are scattered and appear as little islands of color. The scattered type of lesions respond best to laser treatment.

While the *number* of blood vessels in a portwine stain is normal, the diameter of the affected vessels is much larger than in a normal vessel. With a larger vessel, blood flow increases. It's like a garden hose, the larger the diameter of the hose the more water flows through it. Since the vessels are very close to the surface, the increased blood flow makes the skin appear either purple or pink. The color of the portwine stain can change, depending on the speed of the blood flow through the vessel—the faster the flow, the lighter the color.

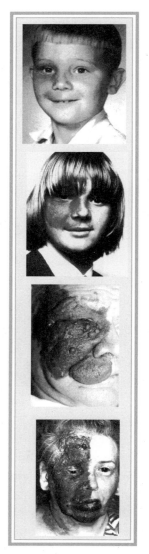

Portwine stains follow a progression. At birth, the lesion is usually pink and flat. The affected blood vessels of the portwine stain continue to enlarge and thicken over the years, and the color darkens. By puberty, the lesion may become a deep red. By age 30, it can be purple. Over time, the clusters of tiny, dilated venules form a cobblestone or lumpy appearance that's unsightly.

The growth and progression of a venular malformation varies greatly from person to person. A lesion can be classified either high or low grade. The high-grade venular malformations progress more rapidly , and the lesion thickens and darkens at an earlier age. Low- grade lesions, on the other hand, progress at a much slower rate. The process of thickening, darkening, and the formation of cobblestones can be delayed until ages 40, 50, or even 60. *It's important to remember that all portwine stains will eventually darken, thicken, and form cobblestones.*

Portwine stains may also cause the pressure within the eye to increase. Left untreated, this could result in blindness of the affected eye. Most portwine stains that affect the eye usually involve the skin above and below the eye on the forehead and cheek. If your child's portwine stain follows this pattern, it's important that an eye specialist check the eye pressure. Early recognition and treatment can prevent blindness.

STURGE-WEBER SYNDROME

Sturge-Weber syndrome is a portwine stain that involves the skin, an eye, and the covering of the brain (meninges). If the skin above and below the eye is involved, it's likely the eye is involved also. Not all patients who have a portwine stain with eye involvement have Sturge-Weber syndrome, because the brain must be involved also.

The effect of a portwine stain on the brain is variable. In some cases, seizures occur, as well as a wasting (atrophy) of the adjacent brain tissue. If the affected area is extensive, the result is mental retardation. But even with extensive brain involvement, some patients have no epilepsy or wasting of brain tissue. No one knows why some patients have more problems than others, but there's a new theory. If the cause of the portwine stain is a deficiency in the nerve supply to the blood vessels, it may make a difference whether the lesion is low or high grade. For instance, in the high-grade lesions, where the portwine stain vessels dilate very rapidly, there may be a *complete* absence of these nerves. But in patients with a low-grade lesion, where the affected vessels dilate very slowly, there may be *some* nerves operating. It's the difference between totally absent nerves and nerves that are present but not working properly. It's possible that patients with Sturge-Weber syndrome, who develop severe epilepsy and brain wasting at an early stage, have a complete deficiency of nerve fibers to the blood vessels that make up their portwine stain. This theory is currently being tested. If it proves correct, it can lead to the development of a test to predict those who are more likely to have a high-grade lesion. Such a test would certainly facilitate a more effective treatment plan with better outcomes.

Early diagnosis of Sturge-Weber syndrome is very important:

- If a child has a portwine stain above and below the eye, it's imperative that an ophthalmologist test the pressure of the fluid within the eye (intraocular pressure).

- If your child has an extensive, facial portwine stain that involves both the skin above and below the eye, and/or extends across the midline, discuss Magnetic Resonance Imaging (MRI) testing with your doctor to determine if the brain is also involved.

- A small portwine stain is not likely to be associated with increased fluid pressure within the eye, or brain involvement, but when in doubt, ask your doctor to order Magnetic Resonance Imaging. It's better to be sure.

Some Health Maintenance Organizations (HMOs) may resist doing expensive tests to diagnose Sturge-Weber syndrome. Show them how they may save money later by sharing the information in this chapter and request the tests be done.

Venous Malformation

A venous malformation is an abnormality of the larger, deep veins, instead of the smaller veins of the portwine stain. This malformation is also most probably caused by a deficient nerve supply to the affected veins. The outcome is a meshwork of large, dilated, tortuous veins.

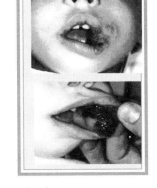

A venous malformation can be superficial or deep, localized or diffuse. Often lesions can have both a superficial and a deep component, and they may occur in more than one site. The color of the lesion depends on the depth and the amount of expansion in the affected vessels. The closer the vessels are to the surface, the deeper the color. A superficial lesion tends to be a maroonish-red, while a deep lesion may show a bluish hue. A very deep lesion will have no color, but will show a protruding mass. The jaw, cheek, tongue, and lips are common sites for a venous malformation.

A venous malformation feels soft to the touch. When you compress it, the color disappears and the lesion empties as the blood is squeezed out. When the child cries or is lying down, the lesion expands, the blood vessels fill, and the color becomes more intense. For instance, if the lesion is on the face and the child is lying down, the color is more vivid.

The natural history of the venous malformation is slow, steady enlargement. Regardless of how small or seemingly innocuous the lesion is, it will increase in size. Certain events may cause the lesion to expand more rapidly: surgery, trauma, infection, and the hormones of puberty, pregnancy, or menopause. For instance, with a partial or incomplete removal of the lesion, called debulking, it will grow back within a short period of time. High-grade lesions expand much more rapidly, and low-grade lesions more slowly. The difference between these two groups may be related to whether or not there is a complete or partial absence of the nerves to the affected area. High- grade lesions expand more rapidly because nothing prevents the vessels from expanding. But the low-grade lesions that have some nerve activity present can limit the dilation. More research must be done to pinpoint the cause.

Lymphatic Malformations

Lymphangioma, hemangiolymphangioma, and cystic hygroma are old terms describing lymphatic malformations. The lymphatics serve as a collecting and transfer system for tissue fluids. The lymphatics collect excess fluid from the tissues and transport it through a series of small vessels back into the venous system. With lymphatic malformations, the transfer of this fluid through these vessels is slowed by an unknown process. The excess fluid accumulates within these vessels and dilates them, resulting in a swelling of the affected area. For example, if the lymph vessels within a particular area of the face are affected, that side of the face will swell up because the normal active transport process has been disrupted, and the malformation results. Lymphatic malformations can involve any part of the body, but most of them occur in the head and neck area. In certain locations, the dilated lymph vessels (or cystic spaces) tend to be large, known as "macrocystic." In other areas, they tend to be small, known as "microcystic." Microcystic lymphatic malformations tend to occur in the facial area. Macrocystic lesions, previously known as cystic hygromas, are more common in the neck. Microcystic lymphatic lesions tend to be more wide-spread than macrocystic lesions.

As with all other vascular lesions, lymphatic malformations may be superficial or deep, localized or diffused. Superficial lesions in the mucous membrane of the mouth are small fluid filled vesicles, sometimes referred to as "frog's eggs" (see picture at right). Superficial lesions on the skin are small, fluid-filled vesicles. Medical texts refer to them as lymphangioma circumscriptum. It's important to remember that these vesicles are usually connected to much larger, deeper cystic spaces. Destroying only the superficial vesicles, without any treatment of the underlying malformation, will result in a recurrence.

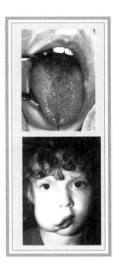

Lymphatic malformations steadily increase in size. Some will enlarge more rapidly than others. Certain conditions such as infection and trauma can result in a sudden, but temporary, expansion of the lesion. It's common for a lymphatic malformation of the head and neck to enlarge due to an upper respiratory infection, and then diminish when the infection subsides. No one knows why this happens. In extremely rare cases, a lymphatic malformation can disappear. It's unwise to delay

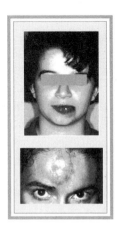

treatment in the hope the lesion will spontaneously disappear since it happens so rarely. You have a better chance of winning the lottery.

Arteriovenous Malformations

As with all other vascular malformations, arteriovenous malformations (AV) are always present at birth, although they may not be noticed for some time. In rare cases, they go unrecognized until adulthood.

The cause of the arteriovenous malformation is due to a defect in the fine control mechanism that regulates the flow of blood to the capillary beds. Most of the time, only 5 percent of the blood supply flows through these capillary beds. Normally, the blood circulates and bypasses them. With an AV malformation, the control mechanism is abnormal: the blood goes in the capillary beds instead of by passing it.

The *core* of the AV malformation is in the abnormal changes in the capillary bed due to the chronic engorgement of the vessels. As the lesion ages, the arterial supply enlarges and thickens to compensate. The veins dilate as more blood flows from the area. The result is a meshwork of dilated, twisted vessels. The goal of treatment is to remove the *core* of the affected vessels in the capillary bed so they won't recur.

There are two grades of arteriovenous malformations: low and high grade. With the low-grade type, the expansion is slower and matches the growth of the child. A high-grade lesion expands rapidly, growing faster than the child until the lesion may eventually become life-threatening.

An AV malformation is a firm mass. When you push on it, the blood doesn't compress out of the vessels quite as easily as a venous malformation. If you rest your hand over the lesion, you can sometimes feel a pulsation. With a very large lesion you can feel the vibration of blood as it rushes through the vessels (fluid thrill). Anything that tends to raise the blood pressure, such as crying, fills the lesion.

Common sites for this type lesion are the midline of the upper and lower lip, but it can be anywhere. The lesion shows an overlying blush color before the mass appears that can look like a portwine stain. The blush is due to the involvement of the skin. In the early stages, an AV malformation can be misdiagnosed as a portwine stain and treated with a laser. Laser treatment alone will not eliminate this kind of lesion.

AV malformations can be either diffuse or localized. The diffuse malformation may or may not be congenital because it progresses and develops as the child gets older. It's usually seen on the trunk such as the chest and abdomen, or on a limb. There is probably some other underlying cause with diffuse lesions since their pattern of behavior is different from the others. Localized lesions appear most commonly on the head and neck; they're most likely to be congenital since they don't extend beyond the original lesion.

Mixed Malformations

Mixed malformations include a combination of two or more vascular components. Frequently, venular malformations combine with an underlying venous malformation and mixed venous-lymphatic malformations. Occasionally an arteriovenous malformation will have what appears to be a very light portwine stain overlying it. Previously, it was thought to be a mixed capillary-arteriovenous malformation. Recent evidence suggests that it's actually due to the arteriovenous malformation involvement of the overlying skin. This is an important point since surgical removal of the malformation, without the overlying skin, will invariably result in a recurrence.

Klippel-Trenaunay Syndrome

Klippel-Trenaunay (KT) syndrome is a vascular lesion made up of abnormal parts of the capillary, venous, and lymphatic systems. It's a mixed lesion that involves one or both limbs. Superficially, the lesion looks like a portwine stain that can be either diffuse or localized. Often, it involves the entire limb, and occasionally the entire half of the body.

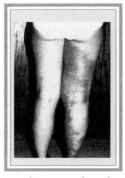

There are some possible complications that need to be anticipated and treated. In a small percentage of cases, the affected limb will grow longer and be thicker due to increased blood volume to the area. If the affected limb is a leg, one will be longer than the other, and the child will walk with a limp. An X-ray of both limbs, taken at various intervals, allows the orthopedist to determine how much growth is left in the affected limb. If the limb is too long, he can calculate how much the other limb is going to grow. He can stop the growth of the affected limb by stapling the epiphysis (cartilage head of the bone). It's important to do this around ages 16, 17, or 18— after the pubescent growth phase is done. Unfortunately, nothing can be done about the thickness of the limb.

Sometime after puberty and before age 30, the portwine stain develops small blood-filled vesicles that bleed spontaneously. A tremendous amount of blood can be lost quickly. *Before this problem can be treated, some precautionary investigation must be done to prevent even more serious problems:* For instance, a normal leg has both a superficial and a deep venous system. With KT syndrome, the superficial system is abnormal and, in some cases, the deep venous system is absent. *Before a surgeon goes in and strips the superficial veins, it must be determined if there is a deep venous system present to support the circulation of the leg.* Without that deep system, the leg can be lost.

There is no cure for KT syndrome, but the symptoms can be treated. Lasers can remove the blood-filled vesicles. This type of portwine stain can be treated with a laser, but it doesn't respond very well. Surgery can be done if the deep venous system is intact. Stripping the dilated, abnormal superficial veins often helps the severe cramping these patients experience. Sclerotherapy by an interventional radiologist is another method of treatment.

◆ ◆ ◆

CHAPTER 5

CHAPTER 6

DIAGNOSIS AND TREATMENT

TREATMENT OF VASCULAR MALFORMATIONS

The type and extent of treatment for a vascular malformation depends on three things: the type of lesion, the location of the lesion, and it's depth. Generally, a *superficial* lesion can be treated with a laser. The size of the vessels determines which laser is appropriate. The vessels can be small, intermediate, or large. For example, early venular malformations are made up of small vessels. Late venular malformations are more of an intermediate size. In venous malformations, the vessels are large.

For small vessels, a flashlamp pumped dye laser is used (pulse-dye laser, tunable dye laser). For intermediate vessels, a laser with a longer exposure time (copper vapor or KTP laser) works best. Very large vessels call for a continuous wave Nd:YAG laser. For more information about lasers, see chapter 8.

Since lasers can't penetrate very deeply (less than 1-3mm), *deep lesions* need to be surgically removed. These are vascular lesions and since blood loss is a problem, they were previously considered extremely hazardous and usually inoperable. Recent advances in technology makes treatment of these lesions possible. The excision can be done with an electrically-heated hot knife, called a thermoscalpel, or with contact laser surgery. The heat from these instruments seals some of the vessels and helps control bleeding. The surgeon needs to have extensive experience in this type of surgery.

Compound lesions first need treatment with a laser to remove the superficial component and then follow with surgical removal for the deep component. One, two, or even three laser treatments, spaced six weeks apart, may be necessary. Laser surgery is almost always done before surgical removal so that there is more skin available for reconstruction. Surgical removal of the deep component should follow 6-to-8 weeks after laser surgery is completed.

TREATMENT FOR VENULAR MALFORMATIONS

Since portwine stains are a superficial lesion, laser treatment is used most often. Rarely is surgical removal necessary, and then only with extremely thick, advanced, lesions in much older patients. *Surgical removal should never be considered for a younger patient.*

Portwine stains need multiple laser treatments. The type of laser to be used will depend on the size of the vessels. The vast majority of lesions have small vessels so they respond to a flashlamp pumped dye laser. The number of treatments necessary varies greatly, anywhere between two and twenty may be necessary. The type of portwine stain that is scattered over the skin like unconnected islands needs fewer treatments and is more likely to respond completely to laser treatment than the single, large lesions. Portwine stains in certain locations respond better than others. Facial lesions on the sides of the face and neck seem to respond the best. Upper lip lesions, lower arm, and leg lesions respond less satisfactorily.

With experience in treating portwine stains, we now know that only between 15-20 percent completely disappear. Most lesions lighten significantly, but 10-20 percent will lighten only slightly. The depth of the vessel determines whether or not the vessel will respond to treatment. The laser doesn't penetrate enough to reach the deeper vessels so they don't respond to treatment as well as the superficial type. The only way to determine the depth of the vessel is to take a piece of the skin. An instrument has been developed that can scan the skin and measure the depth of the vessels, but it's still experimental and not commonly available.

With cobblestone formation, due to the larger size of the vessels, these types of portwine stains will require more thermal energy to destroy the blood vessels. With more thermal energy, the risk of scarring increases. The type of laser used will depend on the physician treating the lesion. It's best to avoid continuous wave lasers such as the Argon laser or the Argon dye laser or the Kripton laser. Since it's more difficult to prevent scarring with these lasers, the surgeon needs a considerable amount of experience in their use (see chapter 7). Currently, only a few surgeons have extensive experience with these lasers.

The lasers we generally recommend are the copper vapor, or frequency doubled Nd:YAG (KTP or KDP) laser with robotic scanner. The use of the scanner will enable the surgeon to deliver precise amounts of energy and minimize risks. These lasers are pulsed or chopped in order to prevent too much thermal damage to surrounding tissue (see chapter 8).

The intervals between treatments is controversial. The portwine stain will continue to fade for six months and, in some patients, for up to a year after a single treatment. If 10 treatments are necessary, it's not practical to treat once a year since it may take 10 years to clear the lesion. Three to six months between treatments is reasonable. This gives the lesion time to fade, but won't extend the treatment period over too long a period of time.

Even with treatment, it's common for the portwine stain to recur after several years. The remaining vessels continue to dilate because the nerve supply is still deficient so the process continues—the laser only treats the large vessels and can't

61

replace the deficient nerve supply. The obvious question is: Why treat it if it's going to come back? The object of treatment is to maintain a cosmetically acceptable result by keeping the lesion from progressing to the thickened, cobblestone appearance that's unsightly and symptomatic. Once the lesion is reduced as much as possible, a touch-up treatment can be done when the lesion becomes noticeable again.

When is enough and enough? Is there a point at which treatment should be abandoned for lesions that lighten but don't disappear completely? As long as the lesion continues to fade, treatment should continue. The time to stop is when the lesion no longer responds. Generally, the most significant response comes within 4 to 6 treatments. Thereafter, the amount of fading diminishes with each subsequent treatment. The risks increase with the number of treatments. For instance, after 20 or 30 treatments, there will almost certainly be a loss of normal skin pigment and whitening. We suggest the maximum number of treatments remain under twenty.

In general, the risk of permanent complications from laser treatment is low and considered safe. The risks of treatment will depend on the type of laser being used and the experience of the surgeon. The flashlamp pumped dye laser is much easier to operate and has a lower risk for complications. Only 5 percent of patients have reported some form of complication from this laser. Most of these aren't serious such as a whitening of the skin (hypopigmentation), a *temporary* darkening of the skin (hyperpigmentation), and thinning of the skin (atrophic scarring). Less than 1 percent have hypertrophic scarring (thick scar). The complications seen with the other types of lasers are similar, but the incidence of scarring is probably a little higher. The rate of complications varies from surgeon to surgeon, depending on his or her experience with the laser.

The use of anesthesia during the treatment of children with portwine stains remains controversial. Some surgeons believe the treatment is virtually painless with the use of topical anesthetic creams such as Emla, making general anesthesia unnecessary. Other surgeons, including one of the authors (MW), prefer to use general anesthesia. The risks of general anesthesia in a healthy child is *extremely* low and the laser procedure is considerably more painful than we acknowledge. There are several advantages to general anesthesia:

- It's less costly and more convenient. Since you can treat the entire lesion at the same time, it eliminates multiple, successive surgeries and the related costs.

- It's a more humane way of administering treatment. Even with Emla or local anesthesia, the child may not tolerate more than a short period of treatment. The treatment is much more painful than originally thought, and the trauma for the child is considerable, especially when many treatments are usually required over a number of years.

TREATMENT OF MIDLINE VENULAR MALFORMATIONS

Half of these lesions will disappear spontaneously within the first few years of life. If it doesn't, and the child has some other elective procedure such as the insertion of tubes or a tonsillectomy, it's not unreasonable to treat this lesion with a flashlamp pumped dye laser. Since the vessels are very small, a low power setting on the laser is used and the risk of complications is extremely low. The lesion will respond to one or two treatments. Almost all of these lesions disappear completely with treatment and most likely won't return.

CHAPTER 6

TREATMENT FOR VENOUS MALFORMATIONS

Generally, the type of treatment will depend on the depth of the lesion, its location, and the extent of involvement. This type of malformation may be treated with one or more of the following: laser, surgery, and sometimes sclerotherapy (where the vessels are injected with a solution that destroys them).

A superficial venous malformation, or the superficial component of a compound venous malformation should be treated with a Nd:YAG laser since the vessels that make up a venous malformation are generally large. This laser generates heat within the venous malformation and causes the vessels to shrink and disappear. It's important that the physician has experience with this laser. This laser, more than any of the others has the highest risk of complications. In experienced hands, it's a safe and effective laser. Generally, 2 or sometimes 3 lasers treatments, 6-8 weeks apart, are necessary.

Immediately after treatment, the area swells considerably but resolves within 5-6 days with little or no pain. Complications include whitening of the skin, (hypopigmentation), temporary darkening of the skin (hyperpigmentation), and scarring. Remember, laser treatment only takes care of the superficial component.

A lesion with a deep component needs to be surgically removed. Venous malformations are the most difficult to remove: They involve large areas of tissue and bleed more than any other lesion during surgery. It may be necessary to sacrifice certain structures such as muscle and skin. A thermoscalpel is used to remove this type of lesion to minimize the risk of bleeding. Here, more than any other type of lesions, it's important that the surgeon be skilled in the removal of this type of lesion.

Sclerotherapy is very useful, especially in very extensive lesions or in lesions involving the arms or legs. It's important to have a skilled interventional radiologist do the procedure. Multiple treatments are often necessary and the results vary depending on the skill of the radiologist. Since you can't cure the lesion, the hope is to *control* it with interventional radiology.

TREATMENT FOR ARTERIOVENOUS MALFORMATIONS

This type of vascular malformation is difficult to manage since the risks of recurrence are extremely high. The timing of treatment for an AV malformation is important because the more mature the lesion, the harder it is to completely remove it. Before treatment, it's important to determine the location of the core and the extent of the lesion. Three tests can provide that information: an MRI, a MRA (magnetic resonance angiogram), or a special angiogram (digital subtraction angiogram). The MRI and MRA can be done at the same time, but the special angiogram is done at a separate time. It's usually important to perform all three tests to determine the extent of the core of the lesion.

Definitive treatment involves surgical removal of the entire core of the lesion. With localized lesions this is possible and should result in a cure. With more extensive lesions complete removal becomes much more difficult if not impossible. In these cases, embolization, with or without surgery, should be considered. The surgeon can block the blood supply (embolize) the arteriovenous malformation before surgery by injecting foreign particles such as gel foam, PVA (polyvinyl alcohol) or another substance into the lesion to block the vessels that make up the core of the lesion. This procedure is done 24 to 48 hours before surgery to help reduce bleeding during surgery but the definitive treatment is surgical excision. If the excision is complete, the lesion shouldn't recur. Although it sounds fairly straightforward, inject the lesion and then remove it, it's not that simple.

There seem to be two distinct types of arteriovenous malformations: There's the diffuse or widespread type that involves much or most of a limb or other structure, and the localized type that commonly occurs on the head and neck. The localized type is easier to remove and surgery is more likely to be successful. With the diffuse type, the extent of the lesion is difficult to determine. After what appears to be complete removal, the lesion recurs. There seems to be an unknown, additional factor operating with the diffuse type of lesion; it's not simply a deficiency of nerves, but some other process. The goal is to control the process and improve the quality of life. In these cases, embolization of the lesion seems a better alternative than surgery. Embolization temporarily controls the lesion but won't cure it. Some surgeons mistakenly attempt to tie off feeding arteries to the malformation which should be strongly discouraged. Almost certainly, a collateral blood supply develops, bypassing the feeding artery that's been tied off. The procedure is fruitless and accomplishes nothing. It also reduces or makes it impossible to embolize the malformation.

If the affected overlying skin is not removed the lesion is likely to recur. If the core of the lesion isn't removed entirely, it recurs. It's best to treat these lesion as early as possible and completely remove it because at that stage the core is much smaller and more easily identifiable making the chances of success greater.

TREATMENT FOR LYMPHATIC MALFORMATIONS

Lymphatic malformations that involve superficial structures, such as the inside of the mouth, the tongue, and skin may only need laser vaporization. Remember, these vesicles are connected to deeper vessels. If a laser is used, the lesion should be vaporized all the way through to the deeper vesicles to completely remove it. Recurrence is frequent, and several treatments may be necessary because it's difficult to reach the deeper vesicles.

With deep-seated lymphatic lesions, surgical removal works best. Lesions in the neck tend to be more localized and are easier to completely remove. Lesions on the face are more diffuse and difficult to remove; multiple procedures may be necessary to do the job. With lymphatic malformations, bleeding is not a special risk—complete excision is. Since it's so difficult to identify the involved tissue from normal tissue, it's easier to leave affected tissues behind. It's imperative the surgeon confirm the precise extent of the lesion before surgery with an MRI.

Superficial mucosal lesions and lesions on the tongue can be vaporized with the CO_2 laser with good results but may have to be repeated.

TREATMENT FOR MIXED MALFORMATIONS

The type of treatment necessary for mixed malformations depend on the various vessels involved. For instance, in mixed venous-venular lesions, the venous component needs to be excised, while the venular component can be treated with the laser. The deep component always needs to be removed first because it feeds the superficial component. If the superficial part is treated first, it recurs because the deep component refuels it. It's like spilling a glass of water on a counter: if you wipe up the water running onto the floor, it keeps flowing from the original source. You have to remove the source of the flow before you make any progress. ♦ ♦ ♦

CHAPTER 6

PART III

HELP AND HURDLES

CHAPTER 7

CHAPTER 7
CHOOSING A DOCTOR

Vascular malformations are unlike any other birth defects because they encompass so many areas of physiology such as skin, vascular system, blood, immune system, vision, airway, and extremities. They can require the expert opinion of many specialists, such as those who practice pediatrics, dermatology, radiology, head and neck surgery, plastic surgery, pathology, hematology and pediatric sub-specialties.

Finding the right doctors can be a daunting task since very few doctors are familiar with all the forms of treatment. A team approach is best with several doctors in different fields consulting to produce an accurate diagnosis and decide what type of treatment is best and who would be the best type of specialist to treat the lesion.

Each type of specialist will choose the treatment with which they are most familiar. Surgeons will think of a surgical solution, dermatologists with laser experience will prefer that method of treatment while a pediatrician will be more apt to try giving steroids.

"If you're not satisfied with your doctor, find another one. Follow your own instincts if something isn't right."

There are competent doctors all over the country who have developed an expertise in accurately diagnosing and treating vascular birthmarks out of a desire and interest to do so. Your best approach is to first educate yourself regarding vascular lesions. Learn as much as you can so that talking to doctors won't be as confusing as it might be. Here are some guidelines to finding the right doctor for your situation:

FINDING A REFERRAL

Call your closest university-affiliated hospital or a major teaching hospital. They should have a clinic for vascular birthmarks or an individual doctor who has taken a special interest in treating these lesions.

If you aren't near a major teaching hospital, call a few hospitals in your area and ask to speak to the chief of pediatrics. He or she should be able to refer you to a doctor who has treated similar vascular birthmarks.

Check with the various support groups around the country (see Chapter 9). Find out whom they recommend based on opinions from families that have been treated. Ask for the name and phone numbers of the families so that you can contact them.

GETTING ANSWERS

Once you have found a clinic or a doctor who treats vascular birthmarks, make a list of questions you have and take it with you to your appointment.

Make copies of all the information you have on the diagnosis and treatment of vascular birthmarks and give them to the doctor. If you've kept documentation on the lesion, take it with you. You may be providing some valuable information that he will be grateful to receive. If nothing else, it helps the doctor to know the extent of your knowledge base.

You want to know if this doctor has experience in accurately diagnosing a vascular birthmark. If you know that your child has a venous malformation and she says it's a hemangioma, look for another doctor.

If you receive multiple diagnoses or conflicting ones from different doctors, ask for diagnostic testing such as an MRI, or another form of imaging in order to determine exactly what the lesion is.

If your doctor diagnoses the lesion with confidence and then explains to you all of the treatment options, you are on the right track. If the doctor tells you there is only one thing that can be done, you can seek a second opinion that will confirm the previous opinion or offer you additional options.

The right doctor should give you several options, and discuss the pros and cons for each one, the right timing for each option, and why. Ask her opinion on why she would select one option over the other.

If you've received an accurate diagnosis, been given several treatment options and a recommendation, ask the doctor how many of these treatments she has performed successfully. Ask to see before and after pictures of similar cases. Ask if you can contact one or two families that she has treated or ask that they contact you.

TREATMENT

When surgery or treatment time arrives, make another list of questions:

♦ If steroid treatment is recommended, ask if your child should be put on a medication to prevent the common side effect of reflux or stomach upset. Ask for a copy of the PDR (Physician's Desk Reference) listing for the drug, or get it from the library (see Appendix 2).

♦ If laser surgery is planned, ask what type of anesthesia will be used. Discuss the different types of anesthesia (local, general, topical) and the side effects, drawbacks, and benefits of each.

♦ If surgery is planned, ask the doctor to explain the risks as well as where the incision will be and what options she offers for minimizing a scar.

♦ Make sure before and after pictures are taken for all treatments. Get copies of all reports on your child for your files. You need them for your own information.

♦ Ask what you can expect from the treatment both before and after, how many treatments will be required, and what the options are if the treatments are not successful.

If you have any problems getting insurance coverage for treatment of a vascular birthmark, ask your doctor if she will give you a letter to justify the treatment as medically necessary. Most doctors will gladly do this.

Don't be afraid to ask questions when it comes to your child. It's your responsibility to ask, and it's the doctor's responsibility to reply. Never feel guilty about getting a second or third opinion. Until you feel satisfied that you have found the right doctor, keep looking, asking and checking.

Besides medical expertise, you need someone who imparts a sense of trust and caring. Does the doctor acknowledge your psychological grief over the birthmark, or are your feelings dismissed? Trust your instincts. If you feel rejected, abused or discounted, you need to excuse yourself and begin your search all over again.

> *"It was such a relief. He kept explaining until I didn't have any more questions."*

Don't forget to use those resources out there. Those families who have walked this path before you will be happy to help you in any way they can.

◆ ◆ ◆

CHAPTER 7

CHAPTER 8

SURGERY

When you make the decision to have your child's lesion removed, don't be too surprised if your friends or family members don't all agree. If the lesion isn't too disfiguring, you may be pressured to accept her the way she is and leave it alone. You can feel torn between that argument and your desire to allow her to look as normal as possible. Go with your instincts. Talk to other parents who opted for removing their child's lesion.

When your child needs surgery, you may find that it isn't available in your area and you have to travel elsewhere. The logistics can seem overwhelming, but they don't have to be if you find out what's available and have a plan.

Contact your patient representative at the hospital where your child will be treated. This is the person who is your best resource for what options and help is available. The patient representative is the contact person for those places that offer special services and rates to families in your situation. They know what help and options are available to you to reduce the stress involved in spending time away from home.

Most cities have a Ronald McDonald House or hotels that offer special programs for families in your situation. The Hilton hotels have a program called Hearth and Home. They offer special rates and services such as TV rooms with a microwave, an activity room, and transportation to the hospital. See chapter 12 for more information.

If you fall into that gray area of those who have insurance but limited financial resources for those things that might not be covered by your policy, hospitals have social workers, patient representatives and discharge planners trained to help you get what you need. They know the services that are available and how to connect you to those services. They can review your insurance plan to see what services are covered. For instance, home care is a real need for the child with a tracheostomy. If your insurance doesn't provide even a few hours of care a week, there are other agencies that can help you. Don't be too proud to accept. There are times when you need the help, and there are a number of people willing to do that. Just ask; it's part of connecting.

Generally, there are four potential types of surgery your child might need: surgical removal of the lesion, various types of reconstruction, laser therapy, and in some cases, tracheostomy.

SURGICAL REMOVAL OF THE LESION

The plan for your child's surgery is a joint venture between you and the surgeon. Make an appointment and set aside at least 30 minutes to discuss all aspects of the surgery. Make a list of questions before you meet with the surgeon to save time.

During the planning session, ask the doctor to explain what type of procedure he's going to do. Will it be a partial or complete removal of the lesion? How is he going to do the surgery? Where and what kind of incisions will be made? For example, if your child is having a lower lip hemangioma removed, will the surgeon do a wedge section or a horizontal cut?

What kind of sutures will he use—dissolving, or the kind that has to be removed? The dissolving sutures are more convenient because they don't require a follow-up visit to have them removed. Many surgeons prefer the non-dissolving sutures on the head and neck area because they are easier to handle and usually result in a smaller, less noticeable scar.

Have the surgeon draw pictures to help you understand or show you pictures of similar surgeries he's done with before and after pictures to show you results. Ask him if you can contact a family so that you can ask them questions about the surgery and recovery process. Most families are more than willing to share their experiences.

Ask how will this particular procedure benefit your child? If you feel concerned about the proposed approach, feel free to voice your concerns. Remember, no question or suggestion is too trivial. You have every right to play an active part in the decision process.

Ask if your child will be given a sedative prior to surgery. Children in a situation where they are going to be separated from their parents tolerate it better if they are sedated. Ask your doctor or anesthesiologist if they will order sedation prior to being taken to surgery.

Discuss the upcoming surgery in an appropriate way for your child's age. Tell him that the doctor is going to fix his birthmark, or whatever term you use to refer to the lesion. Many hospitals have social workers or trained Child Life Workers who help prepare a child for surgery. They deal with emotional issues and explain the procedure. Ask about this type of help if you feel you need it.

SAME DAY SURGERIES

Your child may have either a partial or complete removal of the vascular lesion. Ask the doctor if the surgery can be done as an out-patient, "same day" procedure. Most of these surgeries are done without an overnight stay in the hospital.

Out-patient surgery is a win/win situation for everyone. Insurance companies like it because they don't have to pay for overnight stays, and they're more likely to pay for the surgery. As a parent, you don't have to deal with the anxiety of having your child stay overnight in the hospital. Your child is happier going home with you.

DAY OF SURGERY

The day of surgery will be stressful. Your child won't be allowed to eat or drink anything before surgery. Both you and your child will be anxious. Keep thinking about all the reasons why you decided surgery was necessary. Most of all, don't doubt yourself! Focus on the "after" picture you've created in your mind—the one without the birthmark.

The toughest time is the waiting. Prepare yourself by having something to do. Bring a book, puzzle, friends, work, pray, whatever works.

When you see your child after surgery, *be prepared.* She'll look different with the lesion either gone or altered. The change, while desired, may be briefly traumatic.

> *"I walked right by her in the recovery room after she had her hemangioma removed from her lower lip. I'd never seen her with a normal lip before."*

Many parents are anxious about anesthesia. The use of anesthesia in children has greatly improved during the past 25 years, and there are few negative side effects. Most surgeries require a general anesthesia. An upset stomach or vomiting from anesthesia is not uncommon, but most children recover with no ill effects. Many children have multiple surgeries and become "pros" at recovery.

80

SUCCESSFUL TREATMENTS

Compound

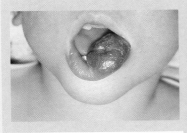

Three month old with a hemangioma of the lip

Six months after surgical removal of hemangioma.

Deep Hemangioma

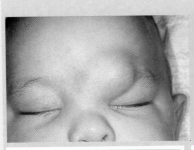

Four month old with deep hemangioma over left eyebrow.

Six months after surgical excision.

81

CHAPTER 8

Compound Hemangioma

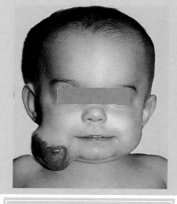

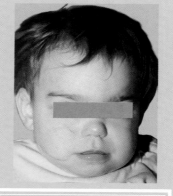

Twelve month old with hemangioma of cheek. At end of proliferation stage.

At age 18 months of age after surgical removal.

Venous Malformation

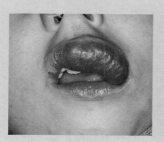

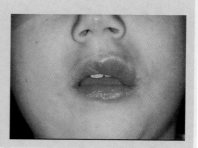

Venous malformation of the upper lip.

After three laser treatments and surgical excision.

Venular Malformations

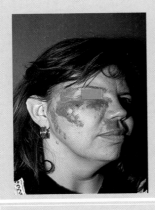

A mature portwine stain.

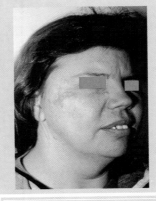

The portwine stain after multiple laser treatments.

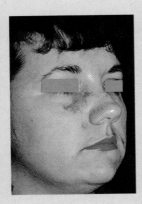

A portwine stain.

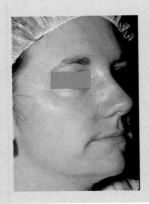

Portwine stain after multiple laser treatments.

83

CHAPTER 8

Superficial Hemangioma

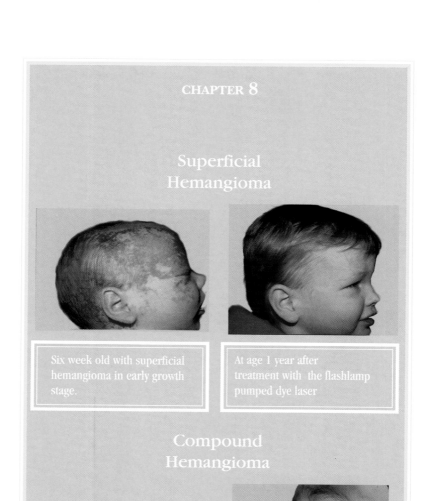

Six week old with superficial hemangioma in early growth stage.

At age 1 year after treatment with the flashlamp pumped dye laser

Compound Hemangioma

Eighteen month old with hemangioma in early involution stage.

At age 2 years after treatment with the flashlamp pumped dye laser and surgical removal.

Venous Malformation

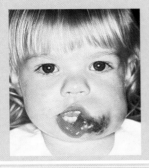

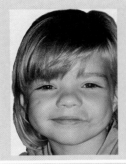

Venous malformation of the mouth and cheek.

Six months after surgical removal and two laser treatments.

Compound Hemangioma

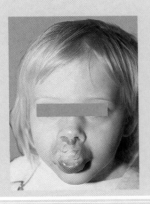

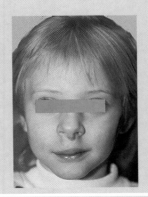

Four year old with compound hemangioma in the involution stage.

After surgical removal. More surgery planned at 8 years of age to correct central portion of lip.

Deep
Hemangiomas

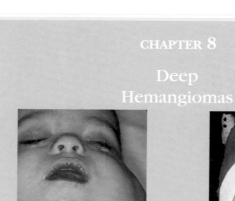

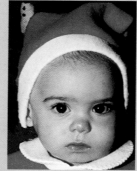

Deep hemangioma complicated by high output cardiac failure in first few months of life.

Three months after surgical removal.

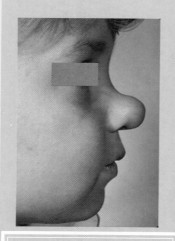

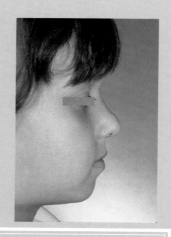

Six year old with deep nasal tip hemangioma.

One year after surgical removal.

Compound
Hemangiomas

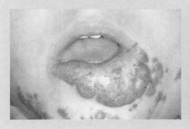

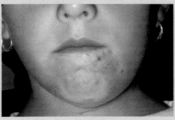

Eighteen month old with hemangioma. Complications included scarring and tracheostomy for 4 years.

3 years after surgical removal of scar and three laser treatments and skin resurfacing.

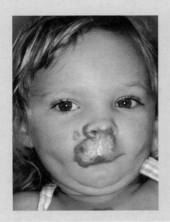

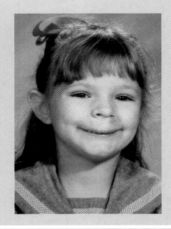

A compound hemangioma with extensive scarring.

After surgical removal, three laser treatment, and skin resurfacing.

Lymphatic Malformation

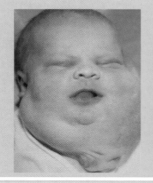

Large lymphatic malformation.

After multiple surgical procedures.

Deep Hemangioma

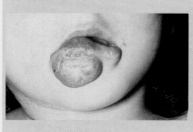
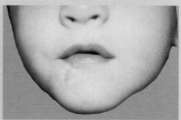

Eighteen month old with deep hemangioma of lower lip.

After surgical removal.

If you have concerns about anesthesia, discuss the options with your surgeon and select which type is best for your child's surgery.

Children are amazingly resilient. Don't be surprised if she's ready to eat or play a few hours after surgery. The extent and type of surgery will determine the level of activity she's allowed. Most surgeries are in the head and neck area and don't require strict limitations. Your doctor will discuss a list of do's and don'ts.

Obviously, a child who undergoes an extensive or major procedure will need more care, and may even require a bed in the intensive care unit (ICU) for a few days. The recovery time may be longer, but the result is still the same: The lesion is gone.

LASERING THE SCAR

Many surgeons recommend one or two pulse dye laser treatments to the scar six-to-eight weeks after surgery. The laser treatment makes the scar less noticeable. The treatments take seconds and can be done with or without anesthesia. You can discuss this option with the surgeon.

LASER SURGERY

A laser is a beam of intense, colored light. When the beam of light meets the vascular lesion, the light is absorbed by the pigment within the red blood cells. The pigment heats and seals the blood vessel from within. The heat must be enough to seal the blood vessel but avoid damaging the overlying skin or structures other than the intended blood vessel. The older type of lasers emitted a beam of continuous light that made it difficult to avoid scarring. The new pulse dye lasers reduce that risk by emitting a beam of light in a series of interrupted pulses long enough to damage the blood vessel and nothing else.

The pulse dye lasers works best for small and medium sized vessels. For the very large vessels, we recommend the nd:YAG laser. This type of laser can cause severe scarring and should only be used by a surgeon with experience in its use.

Lasers are also used to smooth scarred, irregular skin with a procedure called "skin resurfacing originally developed to treat wrinkles. This skin resurfacing offers hope to children whose faces have been disfigured by their hemangiomas. The scar left after a hemangioma has involuted responds to the laser treatment with excellent results. Scarring on areas other than the face can be treated with another type of laser.

WOUND CARE

After surgery, the incision or laser treated area should be kept clean, especially in the mouth area to prevent infection. Vitamin E can be used after the wound has healed on external incisions to soften the scar. Protect the area from trauma. No sports activities, including swimming for one week after a laser treatment.

After Skin Resurfacing

There are three phases to the approximately one week healing process for a laser treatment:

◆ Within 24 hours the treated area "weeps" and clear crusts form. *Always wash your hands well before touching the treated areas.* With a cotton ball, gently clean the areas twice a day with cool water and a mild cleanser such as Dove soap.

Under the age of 3, kids tend to forget about their surgeries. It's a convincing argument for beginning treatment as early as possible to reduce any psychological trauma.

Blot the area dry. For the first few days, undress and clean one treated area at a time to lessen discomfort. Apply one of the following:

◆ Antibiotic ointment such as Polysporin to the treated areas. Use Vaseline if she's sensitive to the antibiotic ointments. *The treated areas must be kept well lubricated to prevent drying and speed healing.*

◆ Second Skin or Vigilon, which covers the treated areas like a bandage may be used instead of ointment. Change dressings morning and evening for five days after gentle cleansing. Don't allow the bandage to dry and stick to the crusts.

◆ When the area is healed in 7 to 10 days, apply a sun protective factor of 15 or greater.

After Pulse Dye Laser Treatment

No aspirin. Advil or Motrin effectively relieve pain. Ice packs also reduce pain, itching, and swelling. A frozen bag of peas or the blue gel packs available in stores makes a useful ice pack.

◆ Avoid trauma to the treated area such as with a wash cloth or clothing.

◆ If the treated area blisters and scabs, keep it moist with an antibiotic until it heals.

Precaution

If she develops increased reddening and itchiness, stop the antibiotic ointment and call the doctor.

To prevent scarring, don't let her pick at the crusts. If she has a lot of crusting, apply a cool compress on gauze or clean cloth for 10 minutes several times a day.

CHAPTER 8

TRACHEOSTOMY

In the event a lesion obstructs breathing, a tracheostomy will have to be done. The doctor makes an opening through the neck into the windpipe (trachea) and puts a tracheostomy tube (trach tube) in the opening. Your child breathes through the tube that's held in place by ties around the neck. The plastic tubes vary in size and type. Each tube has a guide (obturator) that inserts into the opening.

BEFORE SURGERY

Tell your child what's going to happen in very simple terms. For instance, "So you can breathe easier, the doctor is going to make an opening in your throat. The small hole is temporary. The hole has a tube in it to breathe through. You wear the tube like a necklace that's tied around the neck." If it's possible, have the nurses show your child some pictures of a child with a tracheostomy.

The doctor does the tracheostomy in the operating room while she's asleep under anesthesia. If you have questions, ask the doctor.

AFTER SURGERY

After surgery, she goes to the Recovery Room for a short time and then to a special care unit in the pediatric department.

When you see her, you'll notice some blood and mucus around the tracheostomy; that's normal. The nurses clean the area often and suck mucus from the windpipe and lungs with a plastic catheter. The mucus is blood-streaked at first, but this is normal. She may be in the Intensive Care Unit for a few days before being transferred to a regular room.

The nurses teach you how to take care of the tracheostomy. It seems overwhelming at first, but you'll be surprised at how fast you become comfortable and proficient at doing all you have to do. The nurses will give you all the time and help you need.

DAILY CARE

How you view the tracheostomy and how you treat your child is very important. He's not sick and shouldn't be treated differently than other children. The tracheostomy is a temporary inconvenience just as a cast would be for a broken bone. You have to make certain accommodations, nothing more.

THE ENVIRONMENT

The air he breathes needs to be as free from lint, dust, and animal hairs as you can make it. *Absolutely do not allow smoking around your child.*

Humidity is important. The normal moisture that comes with breathing through the nose and mouth is lost with the tracheostomy. It's important to keep the air she breathes moist. You can supply humidification in two ways:

Attach a trach collar to a humidifier at night and nap time. The other way is to use an artificial "nose" that she wears over the trach during the day. Don't leave her alone when using the "nose." It can become clogged with secretions. Change the "nose" at least every day, more often if needed, and throw it away.

The doctor decides if your child needs humidification and which method is best for your situation. Your home equipment supplier provides all the equipment you need and will show you how to use and care for it.

COMMUNICATING

At first, your child may not be able to cry or talk to you because the air from the lungs doesn't pass through the vocal cords. Whether or not she can make sounds depends on why the tracheostomy was done and how old she is. You still need to talk to her, read stories and name pictures. Children are very adaptable and find other ways to "talk" to you and let you know what they need. Sign language can be started by age 8 months. *Baby Signs* by Linda Acredolo and Susan Goodwin (published by Contemporary Books) is a very helpful resource to learn to communicate with your baby by signing. Get the whole family involved. Siblings are especially good at developing and interpreting sign language and consider it fun.

Toddlers and older children need a way to call you when they need you: bells tied to shoes and a tricycle horn are two ways. If you have a portable phone unit, she can press the intercom or page button, or you can buy a one-way monitor.

Older children learn to put a finger over the trach opening to talk and then take it off to breathe. Some kids put their chin over the trach to talk. Some older children may not need to cover their trach to talk. Depending on the circumstances, the words may or may not be clear. Each child is different.

You need an intercom system of some type for nighttime so you can hear your baby or child if she needs you. Many infants have an apnea monitor where an alarm sounds if breathing problems occur. Older children may have a pulse oximeter. Simple intercom systems and one-way monitors are relatively inexpensive and available in department stores.

FEEDING

For breast or bottle feedings, hold your baby in the normal position. Never prop a bottle or leave her unattended during feeding in case of choking. Use a cloth or other non-plastic bib to keep milk from dripping into the trach. Before you start feeding, suction if you need to. If possible, wait 30-60 minutes after feeding to suction again. The coughing from suctioning may cause vomiting. After feeding, burp her well and put her on her right side or stomach.

If the mucus seems thicker, offer her a bottle of water. More fluids keep the mucus thin and easier to cough up.

For the child on solid foods, feed the normal diet for the age of your child. You don't need a special diet. Give her plenty of fluids every day to thin the mucus.

BATHING

You can bathe and wash her hair in a tub as long as you don't get water in the trach. Water play is OK, but never submerge her in the water. Never leave her alone in the tub. Older children can shower as long as you cover the trach so no water can drip in.

CLOTHING

You don't need special clothing. Avoid turtlenecks, necklaces, string around the neck, or anything that could cover or get into the trach and cause problems with breathing.

PLAYING

There are only a few precautions you have to take: Keep all small toy parts or objects away from your child. When outdoors, protect the trach from dirt and temperatures that are very hot or very cold that irritate the lungs. You can protect the trach with a disposable mask, artificial nose, or a scarf tied around the neck.

Contact sports such as football and soccer are not allowed. Unless you watch very closely, swimming and boating are not a good idea. On the beach, protect the trach with an artificial nose to prevent sand from getting into the trach.

AWAY FROM HOME

When you plan to be away from home, make a special bag with only the following items in it to take with you in case the trach gets plugged or comes out:

DeLee suction trap
Portable, battery-operated suction machine
Suction catheters
Sterile water or normal saline
Extra trach tube with obturator the same size as the one in place and another one a size smaller
Trach ties and scissors

TAKING A BREAK

You can't leave your child alone, but you do need a break. Train your spouse or a family member who is willing to take the responsibility of trach care: changing it, suctioning, and doing CPR. Check with the discharge planner at your hospital to see if you can qualify for some nursing care at home.

WHEN TO CALL THE DOCTOR

Your child is normal and will get all the normal childhood illnesses like flu and colds. Take smart precautions against measles, mumps and chickenpox by keeping all immunizations current.

Call your doctor if your child has any of the following:

♦ Fever higher than 101 degrees F. (38.4C)

♦ Coughing up yellow or green mucus

♦ The mucus changes from "bad" to foul odor

♦ A rash or drainage at the trach site

♦ Bleeding at the trach site

TRACHEOSTOMY CARE

SUCTIONING

You have to use suction to remove mucus from the windpipe. It doesn't hurt, and you're helping your child to breathe more easily. Focus on what you're doing, not how she's reacting while you're doing it. The whole procedure gets easier each time you do it. It's not in the same category as changing a diaper, but it'll become another routine you and your child share.

When to Suction

The tube becomes plugged with mucus at times. You know when you see, feel, and hear the signs that it's time to suction:

- Your child may have trouble breathing; he may breathe faster.
- There may be bubbles of mucus at the opening of the tracheostomy.

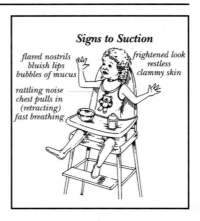

Signs to Suction

flared nostrils
bluish lips
bubbles of mucus

rattling noise
chest pulls in
(retracting)
fast breathing

frightened look
restless
clammy skin

- You may feel a "rattling" or vibrating when you touch your child's chest and back with the flat of your hand. You may also hear it in the chest.

- Your child is restless and you can't calm her by cuddling or rocking.

- The hollow in her neck may "pull in."

- The color around his mouth may look pale, bluish, or dusky.

- The nostrils flare out.

- There is a "scared" look on his face.

- An infant might have trouble sucking.

HOW TO SUCTION

1. You need the following equipment:
   Suction machine with connecting tubing
   Ambu bag
   Suction catheter
   cup with sterile water or saline

2. Wash your hands.

3. Turn on the suction machine and attach connecting tubing.

4. Open sterile suction package.

5. Pour a small amount of sterile water or normal saline in cup.

6. Put on gloves.

7. Attach the catheter to the tubing from the suction machine.

8. Dip the tip of the catheter in the cup of water or normal saline to moisten it.

9. Squirt saline into the trach tube if the mucus is thick.

> **Sterilizing Jars**
>
> Cover jars in large pot with water. Boil water 10 minutes. Remove pot from stove and let water cool. Remove jars from pot with tongs. Don't touch the insides of the jars.
>
> **Sterilizing Water**
>
> Fill large pot with water. Boil water for 10 minutes to sterilize it. Pour water into the jars and lay the lids on top. When water has cooled, close the lids tightly and refrigerate until needed.

10. Insert the catheter quickly into the trach just past the end of the trach tube.

11. Put your thumb over the open port of the catheter to create suction.

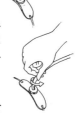

12. Pull the catheter out of the trach using a circular motion; move your thumb up and down on the port as you withdraw the catheter.

13. Put the catheter into the cup of water or normal saline to clear the mucus.

14. Wait 20-30 seconds, repeat suctioning until your child is breathing easily. Insert and remove the catheter as quickly as possible. Repeat the process three times if needed.

AFTER SUCTIONING

1. Rinse the catheter and tubing with sterile water or normal saline by suctioning water through the catheter.

2. Turn off the suction machine.

3. Clean or dispose of the catheter as instructed.

4. Wash hands.

5. Watch your child's breathing to be sure the suctioning cleared the tube.

In the hospital, you're taught to do "sterile" suctioning. After two to three weeks at home, ask the home equipment company to teach you "clean" technique.

WHAT TO DO IF YOUR CHILD IS NOT BREATHING

If the tube plugs, and you can't clear it with suctioning, remove the tube and insert a new one according to the procedure for changing the tracheostomy tube.

THE AMBU BAG

When your child is having trouble breathing, and in emergencies, the Ambu bag can help.

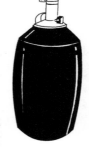

1. Turn on the oxygen, if needed. Connect the Ambu bag to the trach tube by placing the end of the bag over the trach tube.

> **Cleaning Tracheostomy Tubes**
>
> Scrub the trach tube with warm, soapy water. Use a pipe cleaner or small brush to clean the inside of the trach tube.
>
> Soak the trach tube in hydrogen peroxide or Control Solution for 15–30 minutes.
>
> Rinse well with water. Place the trach tube on a paper towel for 2–3 hours to let air-dry inside and out.
>
> Place tube in a plastic bag and seal. If the plastic tube hardens and cracks, throw it away.

2. Gently squeeze the bag between your thumb and fingers several times. Try to squeeze the breath as your child is breathing in.

3. Watch the chest to see if it rises and falls, telling you the lungs are being filled with air.

4. If you're "bagging" before and after suctioning, four or five breaths are usually enough.

SUCTIONING WITHOUT A MACHINE

The DeLee Suction Trap

The DeLee Suction Trap is a portable, plastic container with two tubes coming out the top. It's used when there's no electricity, or when there's an emergency. Here's how to use it.

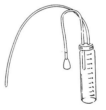

1. Insert the catheter into the trach tube.

2. Place the mouth piece into your mouth holding the trap in an upright position.

3. Suck with enough pressure to cause the mucus to draw up into the plastic container. You won't suck the mucus into your mouth; it drains into the container.

4. Repeat the process as needed until the mucus is cleared.

5. When you finish suctioning, rinse the DeLee Trap in cold water. At the end of the day, clean it with the suction catheters.

6. Dry and store the DeLee Suction Trap in a plastic bag the same way you do the catheters.

CHAPTER 8

SKIN CARE AROUND THE TRACHEOSTOMY

It's important to keep the skin around the trach tube clean to prevent infection. Clean the area once a day when you change the trach ties. If you notice an odor, or an increased amount of mucus collecting around the opening, clean the area more often.

Good hand washing before and after cleaning the skin is IMPORTANT.

If there is no drainage or pooling of mucus:

1. Wash your hands.

2. Gently wash the skin around the trach with non-perfumed soap and water using a soft washcloth.

3. Rinse the skin well with water, being careful not to let water get into the trach.

4. Gently pat dry.

If there is crusty drainage or pooling of mucus around the opening:

1. Mix equal parts of hydrogen peroxide and water in a clean cup or bowl.

2. Wet a cotton tipped swab with the solution and roll the swab over the skin under the tracheostomy tube where the mucus has crusted until it's gone.

3. Rinse with a swab dipped in clear water and let the area dry.

Check around the neck for redness and irritation. Contact the doctor if redness or irritation doesn't go away within

72 hours. Never use powders or lotions on the area around the trach. If the doctor orders an ointment, apply a thin layer as directed.

CHANGING THE TRACHEOSTOMY TIES

Change the ties holding the trach tube daily at the same time you clean around the trach. If the ties become wet and dirty, or if there is irritation of the neck, change the ties more often.

Have someone hold the tube in place while you replace the ties.

1. Tie the ties with a double knot on the side. DO NOT tie in a bow; it's not secure enough.

2. Bend your child's neck slightly forward and pull the ties tight enough so you can barely slip your little finger beneath the ties.

It's common for a child to begin coughing because the movement of the tube is irritating to the windpipe. If you suction before you change the ties, it may help.

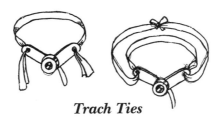

Trach Ties

If the trach tube comes out slightly, keep calm. Simply insert the obturator and ease the tube back in. When it's back in place, remove the obturator immediately.

CHAPTER 8

CHANGING THE TRACHEOSTOMY TUBE

Change the entire tracheostomy tube once a week. The mucus that you can't suction out starts building up. Changing the tube prevents infections of the trachea and opening. You need a second person to help you when you change the tube.

HOW TO CHANGE THE TUBE

1. Arrange a work space next to your child.

2. You need the following equipment:

    tracheostomy tubes —one the same size and one a size smaller
    trach ties
    scissors
    rolled towel
    soap, warm water, soft cloth for cleaning
    water soluble lubricant (K-Y jelly)

3. <u>Wash your hands.</u>

4. Suction first, if you need to.

5. Place the obturator guide into the new trach tube that is the same size as the one already in place.

6. Lightly coat the tip of the obturator with lubricant.

7. Place trach tie into one side of the new trach tube.

8. Place your child on her back with the rolled towel under her shoulders to slightly extend her neck.

9. Have your helper cut the ties on the old trach tube and pull the tube out. Briefly look at the opening area for drainage, redness, or bleeding.

10. Hold the trach tube with the curved part downward.

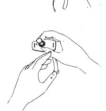

11. Gently ease the trach tube with the obturator into the opening. You may have to use gentle force.

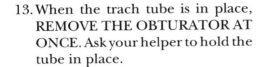

12. If the trach tube doesn't go in easily, pull back $^1/_4$ inch. Try easing it in by rotating it slightly from side to side.

13. When the trach tube is in place, **REMOVE THE OBTURATOR AT ONCE.** Ask your helper to hold the tube in place.

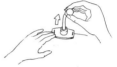

14. Tie the ties tight enough that you can insert only a small finger under the ties when finished.

15. Observe closely for any breathing problems. Suction as needed. Hold and comfort your child.

If you can't get the new tube in place within five minutes, stay calm and try to insert the smaller size trach tube or a suction catheter into the opening. If that doesn't work:

Keep your child with you and call an ambulance or 911 for emergency assistance. If he's not breathing, start artificial respiration the way you were taught in CPR class.

USING THE AMBU BAG

If your child stops breathing, you can use the Ambu bag. Remember to replace the face mask with a larger size as she grows so it fits.

1. Turn on the oxygen, if needed. Connect the bag to the trach tube by placing the end of the bag over the trach tube.

2. Gently squeeze the bag between your thumb and fingers several times. Try to give the breath as the child is breathing in.

3. Watch to see if the chest rises and falls, telling you the lungs are filling with air.

4. If you "bag" before and after suctioning, 4-5 breaths are usually enough.

Ideally, both you and your spouse should know how to care for and change the tracheostomy. It helps to have back up and share the duty. Anyone who is left alone with your child must know how to change the trach if it becomes necessary.

Remember, it's only a temporary situation, and "this too shall pass."

◆ ◆ ◆

CHAPTER 9

EMOTIONAL ASPECTS

WHAT'S IT ALL ABOUT?

Having a new baby is a stressful event even under the best of circumstances. During pregnancy, you probably fantasized about what your baby looks like, what sex it is. After birth, it's normal to go through a type of grieving process for the fantasy baby you've thought about for nine months and the baby you now have. Maybe you wanted a blue-eyed, blond boy and you got a brown-eyed, brunette girl. Emotionally, you have to make the transition from that fantasy baby to your real baby.

The first few days after birth, you deal with those issues and breathe a sigh of relief that at least you have a healthy baby. Then the other shoe drops, and you discover the caveat. Your baby is healthy but has this imperfection. The little imperfection to your rising terror is growing, and you don't know what to do. When you have no control over your child's appearance because of a disfiguring birthmark, there is no greater feeling of helplessness.

> *I felt like such a failure. My husband's whole family is so perfect and I had to be the one to have the child who isn't. I felt cheated."*

Having a child with a defect imposes a crisis on the whole family. As a parent, it's normal to go through the phases of the grief process: the shock and disbelief, denial, anger, and acceptance.

"I thought: this can't be happening to me! It's a nightmare and I'll wake up."

"She had this big red mark on the side of her cheek. We were hoping it was a forcep mark that would fade. I had a feeling it was something more, but I couldn't deal with it."

"I thought maybe God was punishing me. I couldn't believe this was happening. It was just so unfair. I did everything right during my pregnancy. I was so careful."

"When I found out my daughter had a hemangioma, I prayed to God to tell me what to do. I knew this had happened for a purpose; I just needed to know what it was."

Deviation from what's considered normal is not well tolerated in our society. The feelings you deal with are intense and immensely painful.

"Everytime someone makes a comment about my daughter, it's like a knife in my heart."

There is guilt in not producing a physically perfect child. Whether you say it or not, you wonder if you did something wrong to cause the defect. Depending on your background, you might think God is punishing you for some past transgression. Those are easy questions to answer: You did nothing wrong; it just happened, and God hasn't decided to punish you. It's OK to feel sorry for yourself—for a while—as you move through this second phase of the grief process and resolve those feelings of helplessness, hopelessness, fear and frustration. Just don't get stuck there.

It's quite normal to bounce back and forth over the different phases of the grief process. When the sense of loss comes over you, have a good cry, punch pillows, whatever releases the tension. You're entitled.

The real work begins when you come to a state of acceptance for what is and gain the hope that you can find a way to help your child. The quest for information and a direction begins.

"Nine years ago my daughter was diagnosed with a hemangioma. I took her to the leading center in the country for treatment. I remember saying to myself, "They can send a man to the moon but cannot help my little girl's condition."

There are some positives to even the most painful situations. It's not uncommon to re-examine your personal spirituality: your belief in and connection to a Higher Power and to the people around you. You want to believe this happened for a reason and what comes out of it matters. You want to have something good come from both the pain and the experience of overcoming a seemingly insurmountable challenge.

Our friends, family, the important people in our lives teach us about love and understanding. The things that teach us about meaning in life, purpose, and values are the events that change our lives and the experiences that come with those changes.

When a life-changing event occurs, it's common to search for some kind of meaning, to look for and define our own philosophy of life. If your philosophy, up to now, has been, "Life sucks and then you die," it doesn't give you much hope or chance to grow.

The seeds of our spiritual perspective lie somewhere inside each of us. Adversity allows us to grow and evolve in our understanding of our connectedness with others, the Universe, and a Higher Being. It's that faith in a higher purpose, something greater than ourselves that positively affirms some meaning in our life. A sense of connectedness is critical to the important process of hope, acceptance, and healing. These are the positive outcomes adversity offers us. You may find the healing experience encompassing more than just your child's hemangioma or vascular lesion.

"This whole experience had a very positive effect; it was a very unifying experience for the whole family."

YOUR CHILD

Children with vascular birthmarks have been observed to be withdrawn and shy. They walk with their head down and are only most comfortable with their own siblings or close relatives where they are unconditionally loved and accepted. In the waiting room of a Vascular Birthmark Clinic, children are happy to see other children like themselves. They play easily and without fear of being rejected because they're different.

To advise parents to leave their child's birthmark alone and let nature take its course ignores some critical facts. During the early formative years it's important for your child to interact with other children. If he has a facial disfigurement that may frighten other children, he's going to feel different and rejected. It's one thing for a child to see their disfigurement in the mirror, but to see it in the faces of other children can only be a constant source of pain.

It's no surprise that many parents report that their children are unhappy with their birthmark and ask why they are different. For those children who can talk, it's common for them to ask for the birthmark to "go away."

"I don't want this to be here when I'm big."

It's tempting to try to give some kind of positive rein-forcement such as saying it's a special mark from God, but children still perceive themselves as "different" and wonder why. It's only natural to feel different when you ARE different.

Don't hide your child to protect them. Don't rule out nursery school or the other activities that other children enjoy. You just need to do some anticipatory guidance. Go to the school before your child's first day and talk with the teacher and the children. Explain about the birthmark and show pictures of what it looks like. Explain that the doctor is making it go away in time. This approach has worked very successfully for those who tried it. Your child can only benefit from being a part of the class and having the opportunity to interact with other children. The other children have the opportunity to learn sensitivity and compassion. It's a win-win situation.

The silver lining in the dark cloud is that many parents say that the child who endured a facial vascular birthmark is stronger emotionally due to the fact that he or she had to cope with being different. They became a hope and inspiration for everyone around them. It's that kind of outcome that gives meaning to a painful experience.

"She showed such strength of character. Her teacher said she taught the other students a very valuable life-lession."

SIBLINGS

Siblings have their own set of problems in dealing with this family crisis. For the older brother or sister, it can cause great guilt, "Why didn't this happen to me?" They can be angry about the time and attention paid to the disfigured child, while finding themselves constantly defending their brother or sister's birthmark to others. Everyone in the family suffers in his or her own way.

*"When the kids made fun of her, I would make them stop.
I had to explain over and over what happened to her."*

"She always got presents before she had surgery, so she'd ask for this and that. She made the most of it."

COPING

One positive realization is that you have no real control over what happened. You didn't cause it, and you can't be responsible for making it totally OK for everyone else around you, including your child. You can only do the best you can.

You may be tempted to devote your life to this perfect child with an imperfection—don't. You must maintain a balance in your relationships with the rest of your family. Your real strength is in each other. If you retreat into the martyr role, you close out the people in your life who can help you get through this, all of you miss out on the chance to become stronger in the process. This includes your spouse, other children, and your extended family.

There are consequences of closing yourself off: depression is one. If you're depressed, you can't help your child or yourself. You don't have to put up a brave front for everyone else. Reach out to those who can help you work through this in the most positive, productive way.

RELATIONSHIPS

An unresolved crisis can be deadly to your relationship with your spouse. When couples can't connect and share their pain, hopes, and make plans, divorce is not uncommon. The crisis can make or break your relationship with each other. You don't need to heap one crisis on another. If you feel isolated and find communication difficult with each other, talk to someone who can help you sort things out: your spiritual advisor, or a therapist.

The most valuable gift for your child is a role model for working through adversity by being connected to those around you in mutually supportive ways. Let relatives and friends know what you need from them. You don't want their pity. What you need is understanding and support. It's OK to tell them just that. When you need some time to yourself, ask someone to babysit for you. For example, tell your mom or a friend you want her to cook you some meals for the freezer for those days when you have trouble coping. It's the little things that help the most.

OTHER PEOPLE

Because there is so little awareness of vascular birth-marks, the general public has no frame of reference in how to deal with children or adults they meet with a disfiguring birthmark.

"I had to wait until she was 5 to have her operation. Things have turned out great for us; but I do know how hard it is with some ignorant people in society that just do not understand what a parent goes through with a problem like this."

CHAPTER 9

When we first look at someone, it's natural to look at their face. Whether we're grocery shopping, sitting in a restaurant, or window shopping in a mall, we look at FACES. We look, and we think. We notice if people are attractive or not. That's normal. When we see someone who is different in some way, whether disabled or disfigured, it's normal to feel sorry for them. People often react in one of two ways. The usual reaction is to turn away and avoid eye contact. The second reaction is to walk up to the person and ask what happened. It's not uncommon for strangers to ask if you hit your child, if there has been an accident, or if he or she was born that way.

"I've had people telling me things that were highly insulting: 'What's that thing on her face and aren't you going to do something about it?'"

How to deal with the stares, the well-meaning concerns, the insensitivity and sometimes outright hostility of other people who see your child is one of the most difficult things parents have to endure.

"One woman told me, 'She's cute; she'll be fine once that thing is off her face.' I was devastated."

Your best defense is a benign offense: If you see someone staring or obviously talking about your child, go to that person and tell them you noticed their interest. Explain that your child has a birthmark that's being treated. Be friendly. Educating people is the best way to diffuse insensitive remarks or those who are mistakenly fearful you're abusing your child in some way. If you get tired of explaining, make up small cards with the explanation and just hand it to the curious person or the one who asks directly what happened. Most people don't mean to be insensitive; give everybody the benefit of the doubt.

114

FOR YOUR INFORMATION

I noticed your interest in my daughter/son. He/
she has a birthmark known as a _____.
The birthmark is being treated, but it may take
several years before it will be gone. She has been
very brave. The next time you see her, smile...Thanks

Every child has the right to look "normal," and
every doctor has the responsibility to see that everything is done to give each child this opportunity. *The
key to minimizing the emotional trauma is early treatment
and intervention.*

◆ ◆ ◆

CHAPTER 9

CHAPTER 10
INTERVIEWS WITH FAMILIES

Some of the families, who have traveled this path before you, have graciously shared their experiences to help light the way for you.

The stories all have a common thread: the difficult search for information and medical help for their child. They have all experienced the frustrations, the fears, and the pain of a child with a birthmark. Out of this painful experience, each family could identify some positive aspects to their experience, and the belief that their child with the birthmark was indeed special in many ways.

All the interviews were conducted at Arkansas Children's Hospital in Little Rock, Arkansas.

THE COLLINS FAMILY
NEW YORK

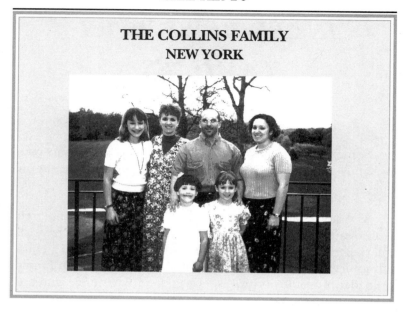

THE BEGINNING

SANDY: At first, Hannah had a big purple spot that looked like a bruise. After a few weeks, more spots appeared. All the doctors said, "Leave them alone, and they'll go away."

When she was born: You question whether you did anything wrong. You look back and think of everything. I always envisioned she was going to be perfect when I was pregnant. It was a big loss. I felt cheated because she didn't do a lot of things our other babies did. I wanted to experience things, like her laughing; she couldn't laugh because of the trach. She didn't cry, and couldn't talk until she was 2 $\frac{1}{2}$ years old.

THE PROCESS

When she was five weeks old, she began having respiratory problems that turned out to be a subglottic hemangioma. By seven weeks, the doctor had to do a tracheostomy. We stopped focusing on the hemangioma because the trach required so much care. She was totally dependent on it for 4 $\frac{1}{2}$ years. If it plugged at all, she'd turn black, and *we had to change it. She needed round-the-clock care. We didn't have any help for 10 months until our insurance company finally agreed we could have a few hours of nursing care a week.*

Because of the large hemangioma on her eye, the doctor started steroids. She was on them until 6 months of age. The first five months of Hannah's life, she was in the hospital most of the time. She spent 32 days in the ICU.

It was a one-hour drive each way from home to the hospital where I worked. Hannah was on my floor. I was exhausted. We were both working, and I was trying to breast feed. We had three other girls: ages 9 and 6 years, and a 17-month-old.

At 10 months, Hannah was off steroids, and the lesions were growing wildly. It was terrible. She couldn't turn her head; she wasn't eating. We decided to try interferon, and did that for eight months. It just got to be too much. She had to go to the doctor weekly and have blood work. The doctor took her off the interferon when she was almost 2 years old. We had to take a break. From 18 months until she was 3 years old, she didn't have any treatments or medications.

PAT: *I exhausted most of my leave from work. My supervisors couldn't understand why I was taking so much time off instead of just doing my job. I had no support from them at all. I decided to leave that job and go to nursing school.*

SANDY: *We were too busy to think about ourselves. I went to work full-time while he went to nursing school.*

PAT: *Sandy's the boss, the executive administrator, and financial officer for the family. My role has changed dramatically, and not just because I went into nursing. For instance, at home she couldn't do some of the caregiver things with Hannah. Even though she's a nurse, she became very nervous. It was my job to give the daily injections when Hannah was on the interferon. When her trach needed changing, I did it.*

SANDY: When Hannah was 3 years old, she had her first surgical procedure. She's had ten procedures done so far. It's been hard for her. Periodically, Hannah would get quiet, and I would ask her, "What's the matter?" She would say, "I'm so tired of people asking me what happened to my face."

One time at the airport, a woman came right up to Hannah, looked right in her face and said, 'Oh my God honey, what happened to your face?' Hannah didn't say anything, but it hurt her feelings.

OBSTACLES:

SANDY: I'd have to say finances, bad medical advice, fatigue, and insurance. Our HMO wanted to find a doctor themselves. They didn't care that we already had one we wanted to use. It took a lot of arguing, phone calls, and pictures. I wanted to appear in front of the board to plead our case. I even used threats. They finally caved in.

Our state has programs for the developmentally delayed. Since Hannah had a trach and couldn't talk until she was 2 years old, she qualified. The state paid for a lot of our trips here. When you're middle-class it's hard. If you're rich, you've got the money. If you're poor, you're eligible for help.

PAT: We just kept plugging away. Our relationship was a basket case for about four and half years. Our whole world was turned upside down. Until this spring, we didn't have any time for each other, time to just sit and talk—just fleeting moments as we passed each other. We're just coming back now. We finally went on a vacation not too long ago for the first time in years. It's the first time we didn't talk about the kids.

RECOMMENDATIONS:

PAT: That's your child. What do you want for your child? Don't take "no" for an answer. Question everything. This is my child; you don't live with this child. You don't know what she goes through. What are my options? Get a second and third opinion. Don't just sit on your heels and expect it to go away.

SANDY: Keep fighting.

PAT: Be aggressive. Pass it on. Get on the media.

SANDY: Our religious belief helped us through this. When Hannah was a baby, they passed a basket around at church, and everyone put their favorite inspirational saying on a piece of paper to send to Hannah. I taped them on her crib when she was a baby.

PAT: We loved that kid to death from the "git go." There's a reason for her birth and the situation.

SANDY: Whenever you meet these kids, you see how special they are. All the moms who have more than one child say that. The kids with hemangiomas are different. Hannah is so outgoing with people, very friendly. She does things that her sisters don't do.

We believe Hannah was sent to us for a definite reason—so we could go out and help other families. We're starting a clinic at our hospital. Parents call, and I send them pictures. I'm able to give the families I talked to my perspective and how it was for me.

PAT: The phone rings all the time. We like helping other families.

◆ ◆ ◆

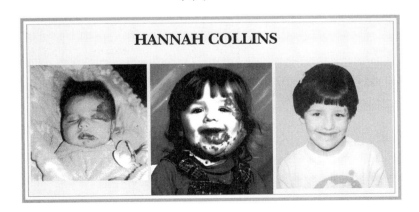

HANNAH COLLINS

THE ARTHUR FAMILY
FLORIDA

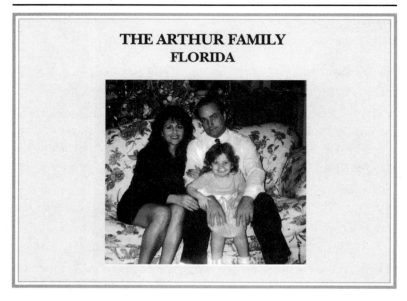

THE BEGINNING

MARIA: *We knew right away Jade had a hemangioma. She had a red mark on her nose when she was born. We thought hemangioma was a fancy name for a birthmark. Within two weeks, she developed a sore on her upper lip. The pediatrician said to put ointment on it. After a week, it got larger and larger. That was the beginning of the ulcer. He didn't realize it was part of the hemangioma. He sent us to see a dermatologist.*

THE PROCESS

The dermatologist said the hemangioma had ulcerated. He showed us before and after pictures of what happens, and what we could expect.

ROSS: *We thought, "No way was it going to grow that big. It wasn't going to happen to us."*

MARIA: *The doctor did tell us that we didn't do anything to cause this, and we couldn't have prevented it. I didn't worry about that because I did everything right during the pregnancy.*

He said it would grow, and then go away; but it would pretty much take a year and a half. Now we had to get used to the bad part that it was going to get bigger, but the positive part was that it was going to go away. As it got larger, the year and half, became two, then three, or five years. Then we started to get nervous because the doctor kept extending the time every time we saw him.

The doctor put her on steroids and she had a lot of constipation and upset stomach. She cried all the time. For the first four months, she never slept more than an hour or two at a time. We didn't know if it was the hemangioma, the steroids, or the ulcer that was bothering her.

By six-to-seven months, she was totally disfigured. Her nose was bright, bright red, dark, dark red. By the time the ulcer on her nose had healed, the septum of her nose just fell out in one piece; it had dried up. Her lip had also become distorted.

ROSS: *It broke our hearts to see her face like that, but we didn't know where to turn. Maria was writing to different people trying to get information on hemangiomas. There was really nothing available.*

MARIA: *After the first year and a half, the dermatologist sent us to a plastic surgeon. He thought the plastic surgeon might be more aggressive with the lesion and do something with the nose.*

The plastic surgeon said it still had a lot of growing to do and to come back in a year. We knew the hemangioma would have to take its course.

People's reactions were devastating. There were times when we went out in public and came pretty close to hitting people because of comments that were made. People came up to the stroller expecting to say something, and then not saying anything when they saw her. We didn't hear any of the normal things people say about a new baby: how pretty, how cute, she looks like her mom, etc. We thought she was beautiful. We took a ton of photos. We were able to get past the hemangioma, but other people couldn't.

I went to the Mommy and Me class, and nobody spoke to me. If I didn't break the ice and speak first, nobody talked to me. At first I couldn't understand why they couldn't at least say hello. I wondered if they thought she was contagious. I know they probably didn't know what to say to me. At the risk of being embarrassed, they said nothing. They might have thought it was better, but in my case, it wasn't. The children reacted to the hemangioma, and the mothers didn't know what to do.

People in the mall would stare and make comments. Adults were the worst. One woman pointed Jade out to her child. He wouldn't have noticed her if she hadn't done that. When I was growing up, pointing at people was rude. If you did that, you had to apologize.

Kids would outwardly laugh at her, and the parents wouldn't say anything. I started correcting them, telling them please not to laugh at her; that she has a birthmark, and it will hurt her feelings. The parents wouldn't say anything, and they just walked away. No one ever apologized.

ROSS*: We had a woman come up and ask us why we hit our kid.*

MARIA*: The worst thing that happened recently was on a trip to McDonald's. Two little boys in different parts of the restaurant saw Jade and ran screaming to their mothers in fear. That really surprised me. I never thought children were afraid of her until that point.*

When we decided to have the surgery done, I called the insurance company to arrange for the operation; they told me they probably wouldn't cover it because it was cosmetic. Right before we came to Little Rock for the operation, the insurance company sent me a letter saying they had information from one of our doctors that we were told to wait on treatment. You could tell they were looking for an out. I sent them an 8x10 glossy photo of Jade and asked how could they possibly say it was cosmetic.

I decided to have a garage sale to raise funds for the surgery. I called the newspapers, and they thought it was a good human interest story. The TV stations showed up on our front lawn.

Because of the garage sale and the coverage in the paper, Jade brought such attention. I was contacted by people all over the country. The community came together and donated money that's in a trust fund for her treatments. *Whatever money is left over will go to the Hemangioma and Vascular Birthmarks Foundation to help other kids with their treatments.*

We think this happened for a reason. God doesn't give you more than you can handle, and there was a definite plan. We don't know exactly what's going to happen, but we know we will make a difference in somebody's life or maybe help change the insurance companies policy regarding birthmarks.

Jade's face touched so many people in a short period of time. The day of the garage sale, people came, not to buy things, but to leave money. If you told them something was $5, they paid $10. People brought things to donate to the garage sale. It was supposed to rain and storm the day of the sale, but people kept saying, 'Don't worry, everything's going to be fine. God is watching out for you. Everybody cares about your little girl.' One man came to the sale and said he'd parked two blocks away, and it was raining there. It wasn't on our block. It was quite an experience.

In two years, we had seen the worst: people had been rude to us, been rude to our child, and we were shunned. Everything had been a bad experience. The publicity turned it all around. Now, a lot of good things have happened. The letters people sent were really heartwarming. Now people come up and talk to Jade and call her by name.

We've been married six years. Our feelings for each other are stronger because of what we have had to go through. We've had to lean on each other. We are very determined. My husband went out and got two jobs. He worked sometimes seven days a week so I could stay home and take care of Jade. Our alone time together had to go on hold.

My respect for my husband has grown— to see a man in public kiss his daughter and hug her. He'd tell her she was beautiful and kiss her right on the nose. People would see him and look horrified. It broke my heart, because I knew he really did think she was beautiful.

A lot of women told me their husbands could never have gone out in public with Jade like that. The women could have handled it better because men tend to internalize how they feel, but women can talk about it. We were really surprised by that. Ross saw me take over as a mother, and I don't think he realized the strength I had.

ROSS: *When Maria wants something done, she does it. I find that very attractive in her.*

MARIA: *We take things as they come. Our relationship made a big difference in how we coped. There were times when I could see he wasn't handling it well. Even though I wasn't either, I kicked in and said, "He needs me," and I was strong for him. Other times, he'd do that for me.*

I couldn't talk to anybody else because I didn't think anybody else could understand what I was feeling. I didn't know about networking with other mothers. If I had known another mother going through the same things as me, I could have used that kind of support. I didn't feel like talking to anybody else who wasn't going through the same thing and could understand. Whenever I did try to, people always made light of it.

RECOMMENDATIONS

Don't give up.

◆ ◆ ◆

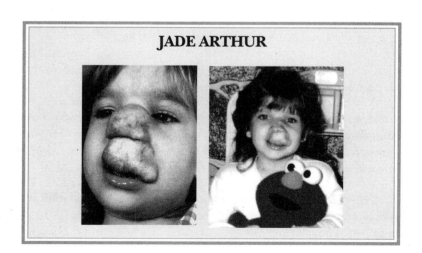

JADE ARTHUR

THE TELLER FAMILY
NEW JERSEY

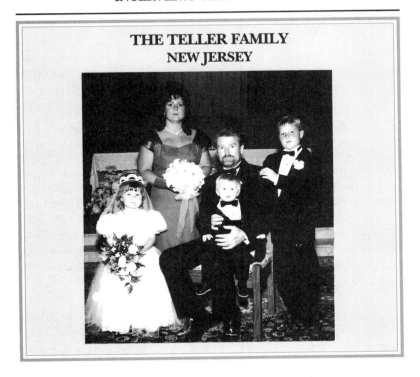

THE BEGINNING

DONNA: *Toni was born two weeks early. The second day, it looked like a bruise from the forceps. Around Christmas, she started having little red pin dots on her cheek. The doctor told me to watch the detergents.*

We took her back to the doctor and he said it could be broken capillaries, or maybe leukemia. He sent us to a children's hospital in our area. They did an ultrasound and other tests. The doctor said it was Tay-Sachs disease and she wouldn't live long. He talked about brain damage. We were trying to deal with that. We were very confused. It started to affect her eye so we also saw an eye doctor who sent us to a dermatologist.

The dermatologist told me that it was probably a hemangioma, and he knew of another doctor who just started doing work with lasers, or we could go to a large hospital he recommended. We decided to go to the one doctor, not a team.

CHAPTER 10

THE PROCESS

The next doctor told us it was a hemangioma and how it was going to be. It wasn't that bad yet. We thought he was going to do this laser, and it was going to disappear. By then it was really growing and she cried all the time. She was in constant pain. We had to take shifts staying up with her all night; the hemangioma must have been creating pressure.

The first laser treatment must have helped because she slept 3 hours for the first time. In her first year, she had at least 17 laser treatments. In between, she had steroid injections in her eyelid. She was 2 years old when we stopped the last laser. Then it was skin resurfacing and lip resection.

I did all the arrangements. I don't think men are as strong as women. My husband can't stand to see his child hurting. He'd be a nervous wreck. I'd have to check him in. He went with me once; when he came home he had to sleep for two days he had such a headache.

The first surgery, I just had to hand her over. I didn't like that. When she had steroid injections, they just took her from me. They couldn't be bothered with my feelings. After I insisted, they gave me some scrubs and let me be with her so I could at least hold her hand.

It was really rough when people saw her… they'd stare. It made me feel pretty bad. People don't know. So many people thought I'd dropped her.

Toni is in preschool. She started when she was 2 years old. She's 5 now. The kids are pretty good. They're used to her now. Grownups are the worst.

Toni hasn't asked, 'Why me?' She's a tough cookie. You worry what her life is going to be like…everything is beauty.

This experience has made our marriage stronger. It was hard wondering what the future holds for her, watching her go through the pain.

My family helped the most. We all got more into my religion. There were no support groups; you just had to try and make life as normal as possible.

In the beginning you question: 'Why? Why did this happen to me.' I blamed myself, but it's changed now. I know I didn't do anything to cause it. A good friend said that God only gives special children like this to people who can handle it.

I was disappointed and confused when we learned about her birth defect—how it was going to disfigure her and affect her life, but I got over that when she started developing her personality. She can, and will hold her own. Now, she's a trip!

They're special kids; they are. They've got something...the toughness.

You realize how precious things are—just having her, no matter what she looks like.

RECOMMENDATIONS

Keep going; don't settle. You know your child; you know something's wrong even when they're telling you to wait. Follow your instincts. Try to find other families. Don't give up hope. The kids are worth it.

◆ ◆ ◆

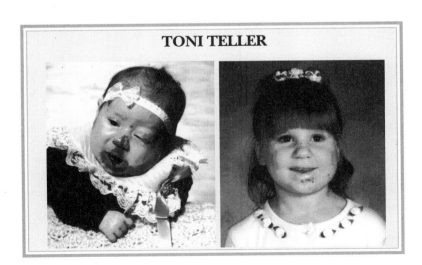

TONI TELLER

CHAPTER 10

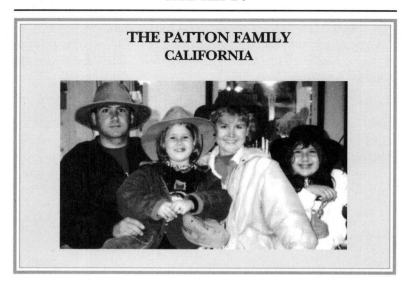

THE PATTON FAMILY
CALIFORNIA

THE BEGINNING

LORI*: We didn't notice anything when she was born, but when she was 3 weeks old, we noticed a red swelling on her face when she cried. By 6 weeks, it turned purple. My sister noticed it and asked me about it. I didn't know what to tell her.*

THE PROCESS

When she was 2 months old, we took her to the pediatrician who told us it was a hemangioma and to let it alone. He said not to let a plastic surgeon near her because it would resolve on its own in time.

When she was 10 months of age, he referred us to a dermatologist. We saw a series of doctors until we ended up at a hospital where they did a number of very painful steroid injections. Not only was the diagnosis incorrect, but what he was doing was fruitless.

It was like finding a needle in a haystack finding the right doctor. Because of the confidence he exuded and the way he explained everything

130

I knew that he was the one who could help us. He said he was 99 percent sure it was a vascular malformation.

GREG: It was like finding God after all we'd been through.

LORI: When Courtney started school, the problems began in kindergarten. The kids would constantly ask 'Why is your lip so big? Did you have an accident?' They stared constantly. Finally, she came home crying and wanted to know when it was going to go away. Her older sister had to defend her.

CHRISTY: I'd stick up for her when the kids would say things to her.

LORI: Greg was always supportive and trusted the decisions I made.

GREG: We were working together toward a goal. It was a unifying experience for the whole family.

LORI: After surgery, Courtney was more self-confident. Now she looks people in the eye.

GREG: We have always had a divine faith, very spiritual. Our prayers and our family's. She's had numerous people support her. Our church and her Sunday school class made a 30-foot banner when she went for surgery.

LORI: I talked to every new teacher. It needs to be explained to the whole class what she had... have the full class know and put the cards on the table. I invited Courtney to say something if she wanted to. It turned out to be an incredible learning experience for the teacher and the kids. The teachers said Courtney taught them so much, and it was an incredible experience for all of them. She taught the whole class a life lesson because she was strong and had such character. She faced life with all the energy she had.

Now I can 'let go' for the first time. Before, I felt resentment toward myself for being too giving and not knowing how to "let go." I handled it by crying, letting it out, talking to friends, and other mothers from the school. Then I could give myself some space and do something for myself.

We've learned we don't have to pity someone because that makes them less. It's been a positive experience. We learned so much.

CHRISTY: *I'm going to be a doctor when I grow up.*

COURTNEY: *It isn't much fun, but it has to be done.*

◆ ◆ ◆

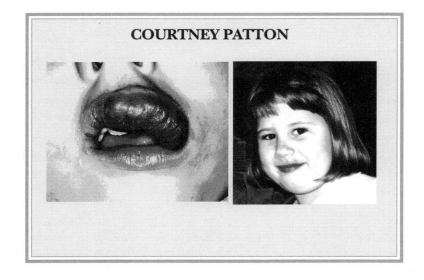

COURTNEY PATTON

THE WYNNE FAMILY
CONNECTICUT

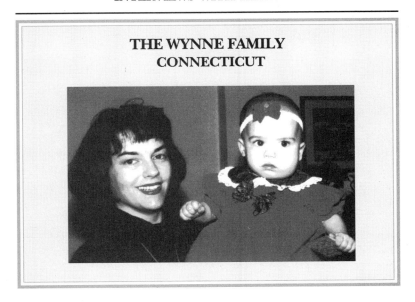

THE BEGINNING

WINNIE: *Mary Kate was born nine weeks premature. When she was 2 weeks old, I noticed a slight purple mark on her face. I asked the nurses in the NICU, but they said it didn't seem to be anything. The doctor wasn't sure, but within a week it turned into a strawberry mark. The hormone they gave her made it grow until it was really large. They wanted to transfer her to a children's hospital because they didn't know what to do. Everyday it was a different story.*

The children's hospital put Mary Kate on a course of steroids, and sent us home. They said there was nothing else they could do until she was 7 years old, and it would go away.

We got home, and the steroids were a nightmare. I called the doctor and he was very rude to me. He said there was no reason why steroids would have any affect on a child such as screaming and crying.

The hemangioma was ulcerating, and he said to just put ointment on it. I was given no instructions to put her on Zantac for her stomach. He also said steroids do not cause mania in children and to just deal with it. It was terrible. She never slept, she was so miserable.

CHAPTER 10

The specialist from children's hospital told the pediatrician to remove Mary Kate from steroids. When I asked the specialist what else could be done, he said, 'I told you before, wait until she's 7; nothing can be done!'

I had seen another specialist when Mary Kate was a few months old. I found out about him because my obstetrician had another child with a hemangioma. I made an appointment to see him. He said to wait until she was 3 years old.

This specialist knew she was on steroids and assumed Mary Kate was on Zantac. He told me the steroids could make her crazy. The other doctor wouldn't agree with it.

She always had a very fast heart rate. When she was 8 months old, we took her to a university hospital where they found her heart was enlarged. She was going into congestive heart failure. I felt totally frustrated. I saw the specialist again, and he agreed to operate.

Some people can't deal with the stress and pull back. I kept going forward. When the specialist originally told me he could operate when she was 3 years old, it gave me comfort to know she wouldn't have to wait until she started school to look normal.

No one can understand how I feel. When people say they do, I say, 'No you don't. Because you can't unless you've been there!'

♦ ♦ ♦

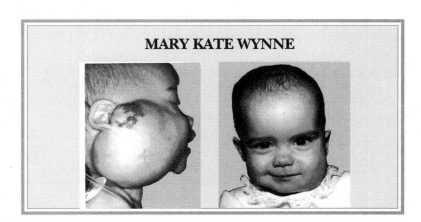

MARY KATE WYNNE

BONANNO FAMILY
MASSACHUSETTS

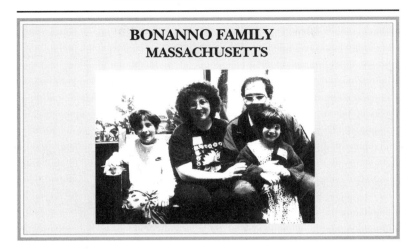

THE BEGINNING

Anne Michelle was born at 28 weeks and weighed 2 pounds 6 ounces. Shortly after birth, Joe and I noticed small red spots on the bridge of her nose and on her back. We asked her neonatologist what the spots were, and he told us about hemangiomas. He said the small spots would quickly become larger, but by six years of age, they usually disappear on their own. We focused on getting our daughter over the many hurdles that preemies go through. However, we knew the hemangiomas would become a sensitive issue for Anne Michelle as well as for us.

To us, she was the most beautiful baby girl in the world. We cherished the rolls of baby fat around her legs and her pretty smile. We remembered how tiny she was, and how we almost lost her. As she grew, so did the hemangiomas.

It hurt us that people only saw the purple bulge instead of our beautiful baby. It hurt even more when people would say, 'Oh by the way, do you know that your daughter has a wad of bubble gum on her nose?' 'What's that thing on her face?' 'You really should do something about that...there are doctors out there that can do something for her.'

135

CHAPTER 10

THE PROCESS

We took Anne Michelle to several specialists. Her pediatrician saw many cases similar to hers. His opinion, and that of a well-known specialist in Boston, was to leave it alone as it should go away eventually. We were afraid it would make her cross-eyed, but her ophthamologist said it didn't affect her eyesight.

At the very young age of 2, our daughter knew she was different. In time, our happy baby became somewhat withdrawn. She didn't like it when other children came up and wanted to touch her 'birthmarker,' as she called it. We worried they would injure it since it had bled profusely before.

When Anne Michelle was four years old, her preschool teacher spoke to us about her interaction with the other children. She didn't play with them even with encouragement from us. She sat alone and played in the sandbox by herself. She was very open about her fears, telling us she was afraid she would be laughed at. She said she was angry and asked why God only gave her hemangiomas and not her brother. We knew we had to do something. We couldn't wait for it to go away. Our pediatrician confirmed she would need some type of surgery to correct it.

A specialist who had treated our daughter consulted with Dr. Waner and we made the trip to Arkansas Children's Hospital in Little Rock, and she became a happier little girl.

I'll never forget how she walked into a post at the airport because she had her head down. There was an immediate change after surgery.

She became more confident and was proud of her accomplishment. She was happy that her profile was smooth not bumpy, Eight months later, you can barely tell our daughter ever had surgery.

We put our faith in God and believed that our prayers were answered. We can't thank enough the many people who helped us: Linda Shannon, Pam Wicker and her family, Cindy Dougan, Hannah Collins and her parents, our pediatricians, and Dr. Waner and his associates who have been so wonderful.

◆ ◆ ◆

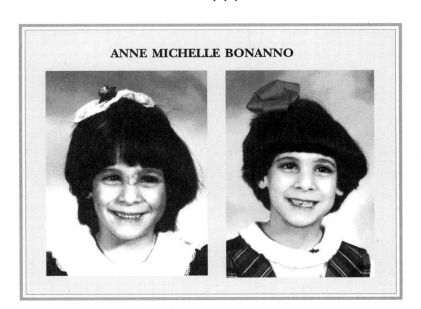

ANNE MICHELLE BONANNO

CHAPTER 10

CHAPTER 11

INSURANCE CLAIMS

INSURANCE

You have health insurance; you expect your benefits to cover the cost of treatment for a vascular lesion. Your insurance or HMO denies coverage. It's not an unusual situation. Many insurance companies still classify the treatment of vascular lesions as cosmetic surgery.

> *"Very frustrating. I was on the phone every day from work. Very upsetting. They were trying to say it was cosmetic surgery."*

The difficulties of collecting from insurance companies for treatment may make some doctors hesitant about becoming involved in the treatment of a vascular lesion. You don't want to find yourself becoming a medical nomad, going from doctor to doctor to find one who will treat the lesion. And you don't want to be forced to leave it alone and hope for the best.

There is a growing movement of parents across the country who have been working to persuade insurance companies to change their policy regarding coverage for the treatment of vascular lesions. These parents, state by state, are winning their appeals and establishing a trend that will help families in the future. Also, doctors are asking organizations that support these families to lobby for legislation to mandate coverage. At this time, there is no national legislation to mandate that insurance companies pay for these treatments. Some states have passed minor pieces of legislation that mandate the payment of treatments for children's portwine stains. It's a start toward a national protocol to require coverage for the treatment of all vascular lesions and congenital birth defects. Since the insurance carriers control the payment or non-payment of these treatments, doctors feel as frustrated as the families over the denial of coverage. What can you do?

The following is a *suggested plan of action* for appealing the denial of insurance coverage of a vascular lesion:

1. There may be instances where you need to see a doctor who isn't a member of your health plan; it's called an "out of network" provider. If you are seeking "out of network" care, find a doctor who will support your efforts. Supply your doctor with information from journals, newspaper articles, or pamphlets that indicates there are new, effective treatment options available "out of network." The treatment of vascular lesions is such a new and growing field, your doctor may not be aware of all the new options available. Share your information. You need his referral to the "out of network" specialist to convince the insurance company that it's necessary.

2. Keep a written history of the lesion from birth until present. Document important information: If the lesion bleeds, becomes ulcerated or infected; all hospital or doctor visits related to the lesion. Document all the expenses related to the care and treatment. For example: If the lip lesion interferes with eating and you have to buy special nipples, keep the receipts. This kind of information will be critical during an appeal process.

3. Seek other opinions that support the need to seek "out of network" treatment. Find a doctor who will agree to do a phone consult. Send her any photos, or the results of diagnostic tests such as an MRI that have been done.

Include an extensive description of the lesion and treatments done to date.

4. If you are denied coverage either verbally or in writing, request a written explanation. Ask your supporting doctor to request an "Expedited Appeal." Call your carrier personally and ask the Medical Case Management Department for the specific steps to appeal the decision. Most carriers have five to six appeal levels. This is where you get to use the documentation you've kept regarding the history, expenses, and treatment of the condition. You don't need a lawyer; most companies allow you to write the appeal letter yourself.

"You have to fight; show pictures, explain your story a million times, deal with incompetent people, see supervisors because they don't know what you're talking about."

5. Notify the Benefit's Department of your employer about the denial. The insurance company may not be following the specific guidelines for your particular plan. A claims adjuster can make an error or faulty decision.

Your employer may be able to help discover the problem. Although employers do not usually overrule the insurance company, they can "influence" the outcome, especially if the carrier is only the administrator of the plan and not the underwriter. Be sure to show your benefit's person your pictures and your diary. It makes your case more personal and wins their support.

"It's usual for them to deny everything and then you have to start over with the whole process."

6. If you have the name of your claim's adjuster, write or call personally. This is the person who needs to see your log and pictures. Send them copies of published articles on hemangiomas or vascular lesions.

7. If you exhaust your appeal process, you may file a complaint with your state's Commissioner of Insurance Department. Some parents have been very successful by filing their complaint after the first appeal has been denied.

8. In writing your letter of appeal or your letter of complaint to the Commissioner of the Insurance Department, there are some key words and phrases that you should include:

   a. The "quality of life" of the child diminishes due to pain or discomfort. Pain or discomfort, as perceived by the parent, can be described by the increased irritability of the child, loss of sleep and period of crying for unexplained reasons. Remember, if there's bleeding or ulceration, there is pain.

   b. If the lesion involves an eye or ear, there is a very real potential for loss of hearing or eyesight when it's left untreated.

   c. List the frequency of bleeding episodes, and the amount of blood loss.

   "We tried to explain how much bleeding our daughter had, but our doctor thought we were just nervous parents, so we brought the blood-stained towels to show him the amount of blood."

   d. If the lesion affects the throat, cite the life-threatening potential of airway obstruction without treatment.

e. If the lesions affect the genital area, point out the potential for rectal obstruction or urinary tract obstruction without treatment.

f. State the importance of having a *skilled* doctor with training in the field to treat the lesion. You don't want a doctor who has had limited training and experience on the general use of a laser or someone who "thinks" he or she can do the procedure.

9. A highly specialized doctor can do a complicated procedure in fewer treatments than an inexperienced one. If the "out of network" specialist can reduce the number of surgeries or treatments proposed by other doctors, emphasize the cost-effectiveness of such an action. This saves the insurance carrier the cost of more treatments than may be necessary. Money talks.

"One doctor told me it would take three surgeries to remove the hemangioma from my daughter's lower lip. When our insurance company denied coverage, I found a specialist who did the job in one surgery as an out-patient."

This parent appealed the decision of the insurance company. Even though she used an "out of network" provider, she cited the money she saved from hospitalization and the cost of further treatments. She won.

10. Some surgeons who specialize in the treatment of hemangiomas will accept a reduced fee for the surgery which may influence the decision of your insurance provider. Ask your surgeon what fee he can offer. Ask your insurance company what they are willing to pay.

11. The National Belle Foundation (see chapter 12) can provide you with a legal letter of support you can submit to your insurance company.

12. Contact the national and local support groups listed in chapter 12. They may have more current information on appealing denial of insurance coverage.

If your child's lesion is disfiguring, indicate that prompt treatment by a specialist will save potential psychotherapy treatments down the road if the child remains untreated by school age.

Make the carrier aware that if these lesions are improperly treated, the cost to repair the damage will be greater than the cost of an "out of network" specialist to do the original procedure.

"Our little girl had a large hemangioma treated with the wrong laser; it caused severe scarring. Her upper lip had to be completely reconstructed by an "out of network" specialist."

Finally, if you exhaust all levels of appeal, find out who the lobbyist is in your state for children with special medical needs and tell them your story. Go to the press. Insurance carriers cannot afford bad press. Good luck.

◆ ◆ ◆

CHAPTER 12

RESOURCES &

SUPPORT GROUPS

Support Groups are an invaluable resource to anyone dealing with the difficulties of having a child with a vascular birthmark. These groups can provide names of other families affected with similar conditions, referrals to physicians who have treated similar conditions successfully, and information on the latest research into new treatment options, and developments in the cause of these birth defects.

> *"My wife and I attended a seminar on hemangiomas. We witnessed a lot of tears and emotion because all of us were going through the same thing. It meant so much to share our experiences and support each other."*

We would like to provide you and your family with as many resources as possible so that you can familiarize yourself with the vascular lesion affecting you or your child so that you can become fully aquainted with the latest developments in this area of medical science. Please feel free to contact any of the resources listed.

THE AMERICAN ACADEMY OF DERMATOLOGY

930 N. Meacham Rd
PO Box 4014
Schaumburg, Il 60168-4014
Write and request the "New Guidelines for Treating Hemangiomas."

CHAPTER 12

THE HEMANGIOMA AND VASCULAR BIRTHMARKS FOUNDATION

PO Box 106
Latham, NY 12110-0106
(518) 782-9637
e-mail—Hemangiom1@aol.com

Linda Shannon is Executive Director, and Milton Waner, MD., is Medical Director. A non-profit organization. providing the latest and most accurate information on the proper diagnosis and treatment of hemangiomas and vascular birthmarks.

THE NATIONAL VASCULAR MALFORMATIONS FOUNDATION

8320 Nightingale St.
Dearborn Heights, MI 48127-1202
(313) 274-1243
Mary Burris, President

Provides information and referrals to individuals and families diagnosed with a vascular malformation (portwine, venous, arterial-venous, and lymphatic malformations).

ABOUT FACE

PO Box 93
Limekiln, PA 19535-0093
(800) 225-3223
Pam Onyx, Director

A support group for people with facial differences.

FACES

PO Box 11082
Chattanooga, TN 37401-2082
(800) 3-FACES-3
Lynn Mayfield, Director

A national non-profit organization for the craniofacially handicapped.

FORWARD FACE

317 E. 34th Street, Ste. 901
New York, NY 10016-4974
(800) 393-FACE

A national non-profit organization for patients and families with craniofacial disorders.

LET'S FACE IT

PO Box 711
Concord, MA 01742-0711
(508)371-3186 AND
PO Box 29972
Bellingham, WA 98228-1972
(360)676-7325

An informational and support network for people with facial differences, their families, friends and professionals. They publish an excellent resource book, "Resources for People with Facial Difference."

HEMANGIOMA HOPE

8400 Rohl Road
North East, PA 16428-2521
(814) 898-1054
Cindy Dougan, Founder

A compassionate prayer ministry for families affected by hemangiomas. Publish a newsletter and hold an annual picnic for families affected by hemangiomas.

HEMANGIOMA NEWSLINE

PO Box 38264
Greensboro, NC 27438-8264
Karla Hall, Founder

A support organization for families, publishes an informational newsletter for families and physicians.

NATIONAL BELLE FOUNDATION

PO Box 385
Gracie Station, NY 10028-0004
(201) 467-9854
Contact: Hyleri Jurofsky

Charitable organization to aid children with physical and cosmetic deformities.

HEMANGIOMA RESEARCH AND EDUCATION

43 Soundview Lane
New Canaan, CT 06840-2732
Contact: Pam Wicker

A newsletter for patients, families, and medical professionals
dealing with hemangiomas and vascular malformations.

CHILDREN'S CRANIOFACIAL ASSOCIATION

9441 LBJ Freeway, Ste. 115-LB46
Dallas, TX 75243-4522
(800) 535-3643
Charlene Smith, Director

Supports the needs of cranio-facial patients and families.
They offer doctor referral, nonmedical patient assistance,
yearly family retreats, and educational programs.

NATIONAL ORGANIZATION FOR RARE DISORDERS, INC.

PO Box 8923
New Fairfield, CT 06812-8923
(203) 746-6518

An educational link for organizations and individuals
concerned with a rare disorder. They monitor legislation,
researches diseases, awards grant money and networks with
individuals.

K-T SUPPORT GROUP

4610 Wooddale Ave
Edina, MN 55424-1139
(612) 925-2596

Provides information and support for Klippel-Trenaunay
syndrome patients and their families.

PROTEOUS SYNDROME FOUNDATION

609 SE Mount Vernon Drive
Blue Springs, MO 64014-5417

Organization founded to educate, support and raise money
for grants and research toward eventually finding a cure for
Proteus syndrome.

MINNESOTA PORTWINE STAIN ASSOCIATION

304 17th Street South
Buffalo, MN 55313-2410
(612)682-1322
Contact:Darla O' Flanagan
Resource for individuals with a portwine stain

THE STURGE-WEBER FOUNDATION

PO Box 418
Mt. Freedom, NJ 07970-0418
(201)895-4445 or (800) 627-5482
Karen Ball, President

Acts as a clearinghouse of information on all aspects of Sturge-Weber syndrome, Klippel-Trenaunay-Weber syndrome and portwine stains.

NEUROFIBROMATOSIS, INC.

8855 Annapolis Road
Suite 110
Lanham, MD 20706-2924
(800)942-6825
Mary Ann Wilson

Offers information about this neurological genetic disorder and identifies local support groups.

NATIONAL NEUROFIBROMATOSIS FOUNDATION

95 Pine St., 16th Floor
New York, New York 10015-1497
(800) 323-7938

Provides information on this neurological genetic disorder with physician referrals for treatment.

NATIONAL INFORMATION CLEARINGHOUSE FOR INFANTS WITH DISABILITIES AND LIFE-THREATENING CONDITIONS

Box 1492
Washington, DC 20013-1492

Provides information on disabilities and related issues.

CHILDREN ANGUISHED WITH LYMPHATIC MALFORMATIONS

16 River Bend
Montgomery, Il 60538-2955
(630)906-9028
Contact: Tina Baalman

Non-profit organization helping children born with lymphatic abnormalities.

THE AVM SUPPORT GROUP OF NEVADA, INC.

PO Box 1261
Fernley, NV 89408-1261
Patti DeLap, President

Network of people who have or have had an AVM (arteriovenous malformation) and suffered from the various effects.

VHL FAMILY ALLIANCE

171 Clinton Road
Brookline, MA 02146-5815
(800)767-4VHL (767-4845)

Dedicated to improving the diagnosis, treatment, and quality of life for VHL (Von Hippel-Lindau Disease) patients and their families.

HHT FOUNDATION INTERNATIONAL, INC.

PO Box 8087
New Haven, CT 06530-0087
(800)HHT-NETW
In Canada, call (604)596-3418
In other countries, call (313)561-2537 (USA)

HHT (Hereditary Hemorrhagic Telangiectasia-Osler-Weber-Rendu syndrome—a rare genetic blood vessel disorder). Provides referrals, support, information and research data on this condition.

NATIONAL LYMPHEDEMA NETWORK

2211 Post Street, Suite 404
San Francisco, CA 94115-3427
Saskia R.J. Thiadens, President

RESOURCES

A non-profit organization providing referrals, support, research and extensive information for individuals dealing with lymphedema.

ASSOCIATION OF BIRTH DEFECT CHILDREN, INC.

827 Irma St.
Orlando, FL 32803-3806
(407)245-7035 (voice)
Web site: http://www.birthdefects.org

National clearinghouse to provide information about birth defects and services for children with disabilities.

THE CRANIOFACIAL FOUNDATION OF AMERICA

PO Box 269
Chattanooga, TN 37401-0269
(423) 778-9192 or 800-418-3223

Supports the work of the Tennessee Craniofacial Center offering a variety of servies for patients and health professionals including support groups and information.

THE HEMANGIOMA SUPPORT GROUP

6349 North Commercial
Portland, OR 97217-2022
(503) 289-6295

The Group provides a forum for exchange of experiences, medical articles and research advice.

THE CENTER FOR DISFIGUREMENT

848 First Colonial Rd.
Virginia Beach, VA 23451-6126
(804) 437-8200
Contact:David McDaniel, M.D.

THE DISFIGUREMENT GUIDANCE CENTRE

PO Box 7
Cupar, Fife KY15 4PF
Scotland, UK
Tel: +44 1334 839084/870281
Contact: Doreen Trust

151

CHAPTER 12

HEMANGIOMA SUPPORT GROUP NATIONAL HEALTH INFORMATION CENTER

7045 N. Concord Ave.
Portland, OR 97217-5439
(503) 289-6295

Provides education, information, and emotional support for people with vascular birthmarks and malformations.

PARENT CARE INC.

9041 Colgate St.
Indianapolis, IN 46268-1210
(317) 872-9913

A coalition of parents and professionals dedicated to improving neonatal intensive care experiences.

RONALD MCDONALD HOUSE

The first Ronald McDonald House was started in Philadelphia in 1974. Since then, the number has grown to 124 in the United States. Each house is independently owned and operated. More than 1.5 million families have enjoyed the family hospitality of a Ronald McDonald House.

Funding for the houses comes from the money donated at McDonalds around the country, individuals, companies, and various service organizations.

The house is a "home-away from home" for families whose child requires treatment at a local hospital. It provides a home-like atmosphere as an antidote to the stress a family experiences while seeking medical treatment for their child.

Each house is different, but here is an example of what the Ronald McDonald House in Little Rock, Arkansas offers:

You are eligible to stay at the Little Rock Ronald McDonald House if:

- you live outside a 50-mile radius of Little Rock. Your child is 21 years of age or younger.

- your child is being served for a physical illness or injury.

- you're an adult receiving out-patient cancer treatments at local cancer facilities.

- you have been referred by a hospital social worker or patient representative who arranges your reservation.

THE HOUSE

The Arkansas Ronald McDonald House has 26 bedrooms, and a one bedroom apartment for long term stays. It's a non-smoking facility with handicapped access.

It provides:

- one private bedroom with lavatory per family for as many as four family members.

- a one-bedroom apartment for long term stays.

- bed and bath linens.

- two fully equipped kitchen areas.

- free laundry facilities.

- two living areas with TV, a VCR, Nintendo, and Sega Genesis

- children's inside and outside play areas.

You provide:

- $10 per night. If you're unable to meet this request, special arrangements can be made. No family is ever turned away because of an inability to pay.

CHAPTER 12

AIRLINES

If you or your child need to travel for surgery, contact one of the following for their policy regarding free airfare for medical treatment. Policies and requirements vary from airline-to-airline.

OPERATION LIFE OFF - TRANS WORLD AIRLINES

contact person: Liz Martin, Brian Zahorik
(314)895-5563
Fax (314)895-5550

SKYWISH - DELTA AIRLINES

contact person: Ruth Ann Robinson
(703) 836-7112 (ext 285)

SOUTHWEST CHARITABLE TICKET - SOUTHWEST AIRLINES

contact person: Tracie Martin
214-904-4103

VOLUNTEER PILOTS ASSOCIATION

P.O. Box 95
Hickory, PA 15340-0095
(412) 356-4007 (voice or fax)

VPA pilots provide free air transportation in private planes for needy people who must travel for medical treatment.

AIRLIFELINE

1-800-446-1231

Funded, in part, by Ronald McDonald's House of Charities. An organization of experienced pilots provide free transportation to needy adults and children.

♦ ♦ ♦

EPILOGUE

I have the pleasure of a friendship with one of the co-authors of this book, Milton Waner, M.D., whose work is the bedrock of this book. He has successfully pioneered research and developed a team of practitioners on the leading edge of the treatment of vascular lesions. This team has consistently and repeatedly demonstrated the efficacy of its treatment of hundreds of children with vascular lesions by, simply, successful outcomes. The success is defined not only by positive structural changes obvious in the children, but by the pleasure and gratitude expressed by the parents of these children.

I felt honored when invited by Dr. Waner to participate and contribute to this book and to become involved in meeting and interviewing the parents of children with birthmarks. The process was delightful, serendipitous, and heartwarming.

In the process of interviewing these parents, I became increasingly impressed and humbled by their courage and aggressiveness in finding the best treatment for their children. To them and you, I say, you are very special people, and even blessed. Each and every one of you has a uniqueness, either inherent or as an unintended consequence of this experience, that is awe-inspiring. Your children are blessed to have you as parents.

—Joseph Brogdon, M.A., Director, Behavioral Medicine Consultants, Little Rock, Arkansas

♦ ♦ ♦

BIRTHMARKS

PART IV

APPENDICES

COMPARISON OF HEMANGIOMAS AND VASCULAR MALFORMATIONS

HEMANGIOMAS	VASCULAR MALFORMATIONS
Hemangiomas are classified according to their location. They are either deep, superficial or compound. They can also grow internally: GI tract, liver, kidneys, adrenals, brain and lungs.	Vascular malformations are classified according to the type of blood vessels involved.

Categories:

Deep—occur in lower dermis or subcutaneous tissue below the collagen layer.

Superficial—occur in upper dermis above the collagen layer.

Compound—combination of both deep and superficial lesions.

Midline Venular (Capillary)— flat, macular stains such as stork bite, salmon patch, and angel kiss. The very small veins (venules) of this lesion are always situated in the midline. They usually fade within the first year of life.

Venular—known as portwine stains, previously referred to as capillary malformations. The venules of this lesion are located in the superficial layer of the dermis.

Venous—erroneously referred to as cavernous hemangiomas. Comprised of large dilated veins in the subcutaneous tissue.

Lymphatic—previously known as: lymphangioma, hemangiolymphangioma, and cystic hygroma. These lesions form from dilated lymph vessels.

Mixed—two or more types of vessels are affected with this lesion: arteriovenous, arteriovenous-capillary, venous-lymphatic, venous-lymphatic capillary, and venular-venous malformations.

COMPARISON OF HEMANGIOMAS AND VASCULAR MALFORMATIONS

HEMANGIOMAS

VASCULAR MALFORMATIONS

Presentation

Thirty percent are visible at birth; seventy percent become apparent during the first few weeks of life. In rare occurrences, the hemangioma is fully present at birth. These full-grown lesions usually involute rapidly.

Deep hemangiomas— may not appear for several months after birth. The skin may be only slightly raised with a bluish color. Feels firm and rubbery to touch. Color doesn't disappear with compression.

Superficial lesions—can look like a bright red, raised or flat patch on the skin, or an area of telangiectasis.

Compound lesions—have both deep and superficial components.

Always present at birth, but may not be evident until months, or even years later.

Midline Venular (Capillary)—Nape of neck and forehead most common sites, light pink color, doesn't thicken with age, and may fade. Forehead lesions V shaped, extend from glabelum to, and involving, the forehead. May involve upper eyelids, alar creases and philtrum.

Venular (Portwine Stain)—head and neck area common sites. At birth, color is pink, deep red at puberty, and dark purple by age 30. The sequence of timing varies. Ultimately, all portwine stains thicken and form cobblestones.

Venous—localized or diffused. Color depends on depth of lesion. Superficial lesions are deep purple while deep lesions are bluish. Jaw, cheek and lips are common areas. The lesions soften and empty with compression. They distend with crying or when the child is lying down.

Lymphatic—head and neck common sites. Usually seen in first two years of life. Microcystic lesions are diffuse with many small dilated, widespread, lymph channels. Macrocystic lesions have fewer, but larger, localized lymph channels. Skin or mucous membranes may have small, lymph-filled vesicles.

COMPARISON OF HEMANGIOMAS AND VASCULAR MALFORMATIONS

HEMANGIOMAS	VASCULAR MALFORMATIONS
Growth Cycle	
Proliferation	*Proliferation and Involution*
During the first year, hemangiomas alternate betwwen growing and resting. During growth, it becomes raised, shiny, and bright red. Cells within the lesion multiply and form dense networks of tiny blood vessels.	Never proliferate and never involutes. Instead, slow steady growth is normal.
	Growth of these lesions is by hypertrophy (enlargement of vessels) rather than hyperplasia (increase in number of cells).
Involution	In some (high grade lesions) the rate of growth is more rapid. Other factors may stimulate periods of rapid growth such as infection, trauma, and hormonal changes. Enlargement of the lesion is common at puberty and other periods of hormonal modulation. Infection and trauma may also result in sudden enlargement of a lymphatic malformation.
By 1 year of age, the process of shrinking begins. The cells within the lesion lose their plumpness and deflate. The lesion turns to a dark maroonish hue.	
Half of hemangiomas are slow regressors that may take 10-12 years to complete the involution cycle. Only 20 percent of slow regressors shrink completely.	

COMPARISON OF HEMANGIOMAS AND VASCULAR MALFORMATIONS

HEMANGIOMAS

VASCULAR MALFORMATIONS

Statistics

Incidence: occurs in 10-12 percent of infants by age one year (23 percent of low birthweight babies). Three to five times more common in females than males. Most common in whites. Blacks and Asians have 0.2 percent incidence.

Incidence—No gender preference

Venular malformations—occur in 0.3 percent of births.

Lymphatic malformations—Ninety percent are visible within two years after birth.

Site: 80 percent occur on head and neck

20 percent on trunk and extremities

Types: 80 percent are singular lesions

20 percent are multiple lesions

Infants with multiple hemangiomas should be examined for the possibility of internal lesions.

Sites:

venular malformations—head and neck most common sites, on lips, tongue, buccal mucosa, buccal fat space, and from upper lip to the nasal vestibule.

APPENDIX 2

The following information on corticosteroids is adapted from *The Physician's Desk Reference—PDR® 49, 1995 Edition.*

CORTICOSTEROIDS—PREDNISONE

While on corticosteroid treatment, patients should not be vaccinated against smallpox. Other immunization procedures should not be undertaken in patients who are on corticosteroids, especially on high doses, because of possible hazards of neurological complications and a lack of antibody response.

Children who are on drugs which suppress the immune system are more susceptible to infections than healthy children. Chickenpox and measles, for example, can have a more serious or even fatal course in non-immune children or adults on corticosteroids. In such children or adults who have not had these diseases, particular care should be taken to avoid exposure. If exposed to chickenpox, preventive treatment with varicella zoster immune globulin (VZIG) may be indicated. If exposed to measles, preventive treatment with pooled intravenous immunoglobulin (IVIG) may be indicated.

PRECAUTIONS

Patients who are on immunosuppressant doses of corticosteroids should be warned to avoid exposure to chickenpox or measles. Patients should also be advised that if they are exposed, medical advice should be sought without delay.

The lowest possible dose of corticosteroid should be used to control the condition under treatment, and when reduction in dosage is possible, the reduction should be gradual. Psychic derangement may appear when corticosteroids are used, ranging from euphoria, insomnia, mood swings, personality changes, and severe depression to frankly psychotic manifestations. Also, existing emotional instability or psychotic tendencies may be aggravated by corticosteroids.

Growth and development of infants and children on prolonged corticosteroid therapy should be carefully observed.

POSSIBLE ADVERSE REACTIONS

edema (swelling)

congestive heart failure

loss of muscle mass

peptic ulcer with possible perforation (hole in stomach lining) and hemorrhage (bleeding)

abdominal distension

thin fragile skin

petechiae (small hemorrhagic spots) and ecchymoses (bruising)

facial erythema (redness)

convulsions

suppression of growth in children (growth retardation or failure to thrive)

APPENDIX 3

BIBLIOGRAPHY &
REFERENCES

Ashinoff R. and Geronemus RG: Capillary hemangiomas and treatment with the flashlamp pumped pulsed dye laser: Prospective analysis. *J. Pediatr.*, 4:555-560, 1992.

Enjolras O, Riche MD, Merland JJ, et al: Management of alarming hemangiomas in infancy: A review of 25 cases. *Pediatrics,* 85:491-498, 1990.

Ezekowitz RAB, Mulliken JB, and Folkman J: Interferon Alfa-2a therapy for life-threatening hemangiomas of infancy. *N. Engl. J. Med.* 326:1456-63, 1992.

Ezekowitz RAB: Pharmacologic therapy for endangering hemangiomas. *Current Opinion in Dermatol.* 109-113, 1995.

Sadan N, Wolach B: Treatment of hemangiomas of infants with high doses of prednisone. *J. Ped.* 128:141-146, 1996.

Finn MC, Glowacki, and Mulliken JB: Congenital vascular lesions: Clinical application of a new classification. *J. Ped. Surg.* 18:894, 1983.

Guyer DR, Tiedeman J, Yannuzzi LA, et al: Interferon-associated retinopathy. *Arch Opthalmol,* 111:350-356, 1993.

Kunkel EJ, Zager RP, Hausman CL, et. al.:An interdisciplinary group for parents of children with hemangiomas. *Psychosomatics.* 35(6):524-532, 1994

Lister W.A: The Natural history of strawberry naevai, *Lancet*, 1:1429-1434, 1938.

Mulliken JB: Vascular malformations of the head and neck, in Mulliken JB, Young AE (eds): *Vascular Birthmarks: Hemangiomas and Vascular Malformations.* WB Saunders Co., Philadelphia, Pa., 1988.

Mulliken JB, and Glowacki J: Hemangiomas and vascular malformations in infants and children: A classification based on endothelial characteristics. *Plast. Reconstr. Surg.* 69:412, 1982.

Shakin Kunkel EJ, Zager RP, Hausman CL, & Rabinowitz LG: An interdisciplinary group for parents of children with hemangiomas. *Psychosomatics* 35:524, 1994.

Vesikari T, Nuutila A, Cantell K: Neurologic sequelae following interferon therapy of juvenile laryngeal papilloma. *Acta Paediatr Scand,* 77:619-622, 1988.

Waner M, Suen JY: Treatment of hemangiomas of the head and neck. *Laryngoscope*, 102:1123-1132, 1992.

Waner M, Suen JY, Dinehart S, Mallory SB: Laser photocoagulation of superficial proliferating hemangiomas. *Journal of Dermatology/Surgery/Oncology*, 21:1-4, 1994.

Waner M, Suen JY: Advances in the management of congenital vascular lesions of the head and neck. *Advances in Otolaryngology*, 10:31-54, 1996.

Wheeland RG: Treatment of portwine stains for the 1990s. *J. Dermatol Surg Oncol.* 19:348-356, 1993.

Index

TO ORDER ADDITIONAL COPIES
18.95 per copy

- -

ORDER FORM

Add $3.50 postage and handling for one book order, $4.50 for two books, and $5.50 for three books.

NAME_____

TITLE_____

ADDRESS_____

CITY_____STATE_____ ZIP_____

PHONE_____

Please send me _____ copies of

Birthmarks: A Guide to Hemangiomas and Vascular Malformations

My check or money order for $_____enclosed

- -

MAIL ORDER FORM TO:

Women's Health Publishing Inc.
1176 Angela Court, Ste. 103
Minden, NV 89423

OR CALL TOLL FREE: **1-888-235-7947**